Imaging of Sports Injuries

Arnold Williams, F.R.C.R., F.R.C.S.
Consultant Radiologist
Cardiff Royal Infirmary

Roger Evans, F.R.C.P.
Consultant in Accident & Emergency Medicine
Cardiff Royal Infirmary

Paul D. Shirley, M.D., P.A.
Consultant Orthopaedic Surgeon
Jacksonville, Florida

Baillière Tindall
LONDON PHILADELPHIA TORONTO SYDNEY TOKYO

Baillière Tindall 24-28 Oval Road
W. B. Saunders London NW1 7DX, England

The Curtis Center
Independence Square West
Philadelphia, PA 19106-3399, USA

1 Goldthorne Avenue
Toronto, Ontario M8Z 5T9, Canada

Harcourt Brace Jovanovich Group (Australia) Pty Ltd
32-52 Smidmore Street
Marrickville, NSW 2204, Australia

Harcourt Brace Jovanovich Japan Inc.
Ichibancho Central Building, 22-1 Ichibancho
Chiyoda-ku, Tokyo 102, Japan

British Library Cataloguing in Publication Data

Williams, L. A.
  Imaging sports injuries
  1. Sports and games. Injuries.
  Diagnosis. Imaging.
  I. Title.   II. Evans, R. C.
  III. Shirley, P. D.
  617'.1027

  ISBN 0-7020-1368-4

Typeset by Dobbie Typesetting Limited, Plymouth, Devon.
Printed in Great Britain by
Thomson Litho Ltd, East Kilbride, Scotland

Contents

Preface

The past three or four decades have seen immense changes in sports and allied leisure activities. The number of sports open to general participation has multiplied and along with this have gone major developments in the provision of sporting facilities. An increase in prosperity and a greater amount of leisure time together with an urge to maintain fitness has resulted in many more people continuing or restarting athletic activities beyond their days in full-time education.

Thirty years ago the number of participants involved in tae-kwondo or karate in the Western world would have been negligible, but today many thousands of people are active in these and other martial arts. Some events such as the triathlon were unheard of in the 1950s, as were activities such as windsurfing or skateboarding, which are common today. Sports such as squash have seen a major increase in the number of participants and there has been a positive explosion in the size of the fields for marathons and half-marathons.

There have always been 'high risk' sports such as mountaineering and skiing but in recent years many others have appeared and become popular including parachuting, hang-gliding and cross-country racing on a variety of all-terrain vehicles. This has resulted in an increase in the number of serious sports-related injuries, particularly to regions such as the head, neck and spine.

Whilst there has been this surge in the number of 'amateur' sportsmen and women, the world of the 'professional' athlete, paid or unpaid, has undergone equally radical changes. In the 1980s competition is fiercer and the financial rewards are far greater than ever before; consequently the degree of dedication required to reach the very top is now all-consuming. The day of the Corinthian has passed and the time when those selected for an international team turned up with their kit on a Saturday morning to play in the afternoon has long gone. Sport at the top is now a year round, full-time occupation.

Rather tardily perhaps, along with this growth in the popularity of sport there has been an increased interest amongst some members of the medical and allied professions in the problems produced for athletes by their exertions. Immense work has been done by members of the various associations of sports medicine in many countries to foster interest amongst their fellow practitioners in sports-related problems and this has often been against a tide of feeling that regards such damage as self-inflicted, an injury that can be best 'cured' by the patient giving up his or her sport.

Most doctors who are not involved in the treatment of athletes have little idea of how much time and effort top-line performers put into their training; 20 to 30 hours a week in the pool or 120 miles a week of road work is not uncommon, and this may be in association with an attempt to hold down a job or to keep up with a full-time academic course.

Whilst we accept that some of the injuries sustained by athletes, such as torn menisci, do occur in the general population, other injuries are specifically related to the heavy physical demands that athletic men and women place upon their bodies. In their drive to succeed, many younger athletes sustain injuries to immature skeletons which give rise to problems both immediately and in later life. The current vogue for increased activity in people aged over 40 years, in the belief that this benefits the cardiovascular system, also produces difficulties. In both the 'paediatric' and 'geriatric' athlete, injuries occur in which the diagnosis may remain obscure for long periods.

Arriving at a diagnosis in these patients has been made easier by the advances in imaging techniques that have appeared in recent years. The plain radiograph may now be supplemented by isotope bone scanning (scintigraphy), thermography, xeroradiography, computerized tomography (CT), high quality ultrasound (US), and most recently magnetic resonance imaging (MRI).

In this book we have illustrated the conditions that we see in our sports medicine practice, including pictures of some classical problems and one or two more unusual injuries, and we have also drawn attention to some of the pitfalls that lie in wait for the unwary. We are aware that athletes can sustain any of the bony injuries that are described in large comprehensive textbooks of orthopaedics, but for us to have included all of these would have rendered this volume unmanageable.

We should like to express our appreciation of the work of Mrs Janet Braddon in producing the manuscript draft and Mr Keith Bellamy for his work on the illustrations. Our thanks, also, must go to Dr Basil Strickland, Dr Francis Ring, Mr Patrick England and Dr Margaret Hourihan who very kindly allowed us to reproduce illustrations from cases under their care.

1 Skull and Facial Bones

Head and facial injuries occur mostly in contact sports and are usually nothing more than bruises or lacerations, sometimes accompanied by a mild concussive injury to the brain. The commonest fractures that we see are to the nasal and cheek bones as the vault of the skull is a particularly strong structure. Where the skull is fractured it is commonly in a linear fashion as can be seen in Figure 1.1 which is the lateral view showing a fracture to the right parietal in a 19-year-old soccer player.

Depressed fractures are more significant and more commonly need neurosurgical intervention. They can often be diagnosed clinically, as indeed was the injury illustrated in Figure 1.2, a localized view of the right side of the skull demonstrating a large depressed fracture sustained in a fall from an all-terrain vehicle.

Smaller depressed fractures can readily be missed on plain films although their presence may be suspected by the demonstration of a small area of increased density which is produced by the overlapping of the bone edges. Where such an abnormality is noted the fracture may be more easily demonstrated by taking oblique views of the vault in an attempt to place the fractured area on the 'sky-line' as has been done in Figure 1.3 which illustrates such an injury sustained by a gymnast.

In more difficult cases a CT scan will demonstrate the lesion clearly and this is now probably the investigation of choice. Figure 1.4 shows a depressed fracture with intracranial bone fragments, an injury sustained by a 43-year-old golfer. Such a scan may also demonstrate an intracranial communication with a superficial wound and will highlight any intracranial collections of air as shown in Figure 1.5 which is an injury that will certainly need surgical intervention.

Injuries to the underlying brain and intracranial vasculature are of far more importance than straightforward fractures, and significant intracranial damage may be produced without a fracture being present. Accurate neurological assessment of the patient immediately after the injury and subsequently is vital, and the investigation of choice at present is a CT scan which would demonstrate any collection of intracranial blood. Of particular importance is the early detection of subdural or extradural haematomas (Figure 1.6) which need to be evacuated. This scan demonstrates a large subdural pool in a 38-year-old horsewoman, sustained when she was thrown. CT scanning readily demonstrates the abnormalities just described, but the newer technique of magnetic resonance imaging (MRI) is useful for detecting more subtle damage to the brain itself.

Repeated head injuries, for instance in boxers, produce minor intracranial damage and this can eventually result in a chronic progressive post-traumatic encephalopathy with scarring of the brain and later cerebral atrophy. One of the earliest radiological signs of this damage is the development of a cavum septum pellucidum as shown in Figures 1.7 and 1.8 which are illustrations of CT scans of the head of a 25-year-old heavyweight boxer whose career was ended by these findings.

More gross examples of cerebral atrophy are usually found in older boxers (Figure 1.9) who in the past have been allowed to fight two or three hundred bouts or more, sometimes outside their weight limits. This is an outdated practice which would no longer be tolerated by the boxing boards of control.

Fractures of the nasal bones are normally easily diagnosed due to their subcutaneous position. They may not require any treatment unless there is marked displacement and deformity or the nasal airway is significantly compromised. As nasal injuries are so frequent in contact sports it is often better to postpone definitive treatment until after the player's career has ended.

Depressed fractures of the zygomatic arch should also be readily diagnosed clinically, although soft tissue swelling which occurs within minutes may disguise the underlying deformity. A clue to the presence of such a fracture may be found in Figure 1.10 where the patient had difficulty in opening his mouth due to impingement of the mandible upon the depressed zygomatic arch. This injury was sustained by a 34-year-old rugby player, and required elevation and fixation. Fractures to the lower part of the orbit can be difficult to pick out radiologically, although clinically anaesthesia in the distribution of the infraorbital nerve or an ophthalmoplegia with diplopia almost always indicate a fracture, as does the demonstration of air around the eye in the absence of any penetrating injury. Figure 1.11 illustrates this sign which points to a fracture communicating with one of the adjacent sinuses. This injury was caused by a blow to the face sustained by a 31-year-old rugby player.

Direct trauma to the eye by a squash ball can lead to uniocular blindness, although less serious injuries occasionally result in the soft tissues contained in the orbit being forced inferiorly through the floor which is the weakest part of that structure. This situation is seen in Figure 1.12; herniation of the orbital contents into the antrum shows as a soft tissue mass together with a collection of blood.

Fractures of the mandible are quite common and the clinical picture

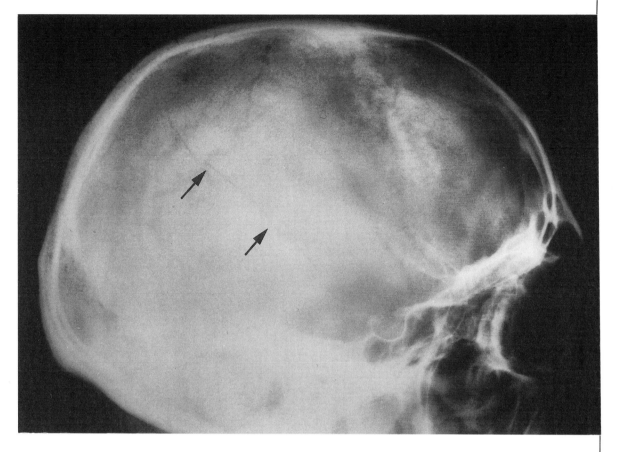

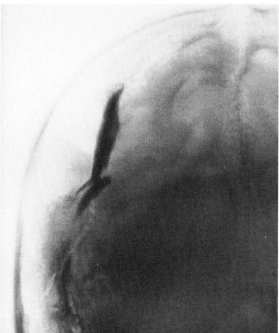

Figure 1.1. (Above). Lateral X-ray of the skull showing a long linear fracture of the parietal bone.

Figure 1.2. (Left). Occipitomental view localizing on the right side, demonstrating a large depressed fracture.

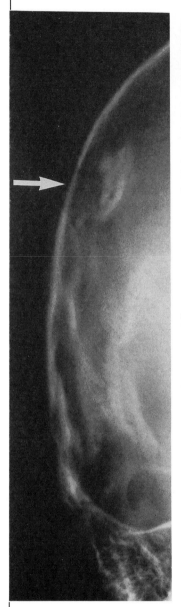

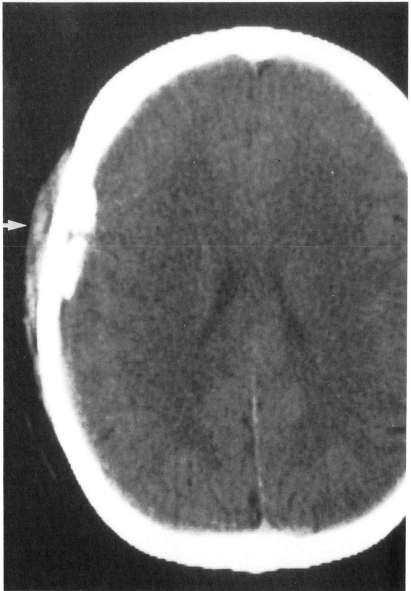

Figure 1.3. (Above left). Oblique view of the skull showing a small depressed fracture seen as an area of increased sclerosis in a double line.

Figure 1.4. (Above right). CT scan of a head demonstrating a large depressed fracture with some intracranial bone fragments.

is usually clear-cut. However, the whole of the bone must be inspected as it is not unusual for a fracture of the body of the mandible on one side to be associated with a fracture of the neck of the condyle on the other (Figures 1.13 and 1.14); the latter fracture is easily missed.

Direct blows to the mandible may drive the condyle into the temporomandibular joint, resulting in damage to the meniscus. Further investigation may require arthrography of the temporomandibular joint to demonstrate intra-articular structures. There are reports of the satisfactory use of CT and MRI in the investigation of lesions at this site, but we have little experience of the techniques.

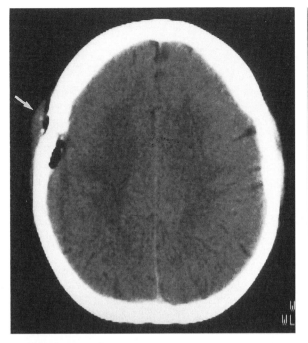

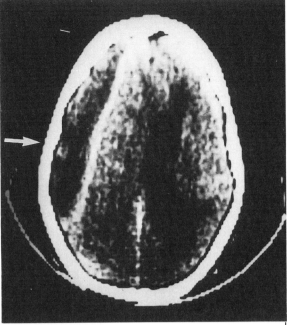

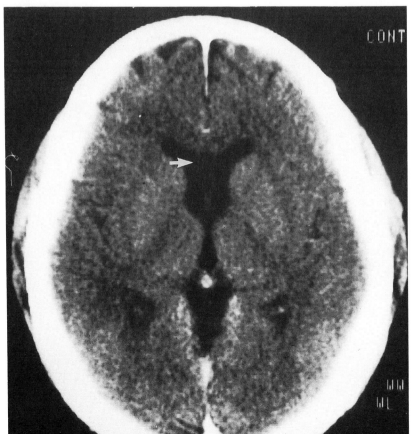

Figure 1.5. (Above left). CT scan of the skull of a patient with a compound fracture. Note the air in the soft tissues and also the intracranial collection of air.

Figure 1.6. (Above right). CT scan of the head demonstrating a large subdural haematoma.

Figure 1.7. (Left). CT scan of the brain with demonstration of a small cavum septum pellucidum.

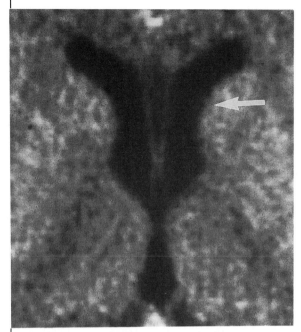

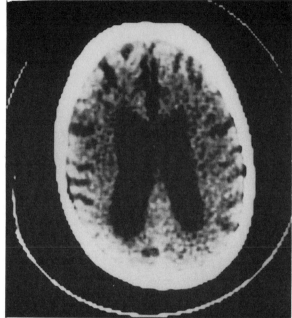

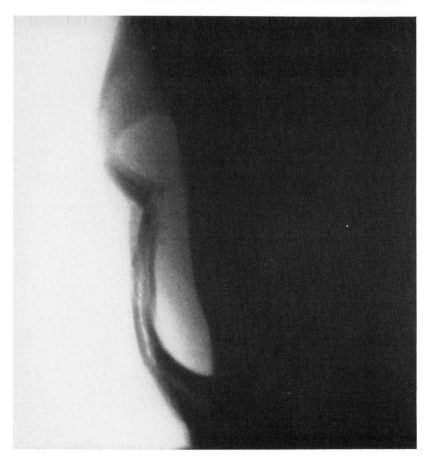

Figure 1.8. (Above left). Magnified view of Figure 1.7 showing the cavum more clearly.

Figure 1.9. (Above right). CT scan of the brain showing markedly dilated ventricles and enlarged sulci due to gross cerebral atrophy.

Figure 1.10. (Right). Oblique 'sky-line' view demonstrating the zygomatic arch which is fractured and depressed.

Figure 1.11. (Facing top). Occipitomental view of the orbits showing air in the right orbit due to a non-visualized fracture extending into one of the sinuses.

Figure 1.12. (Facing bottom). Occipitomental view of the orbits demonstrating a blow-out fracture of the floor of the right orbit with herniation of orbital tissue into the right antrum.

6

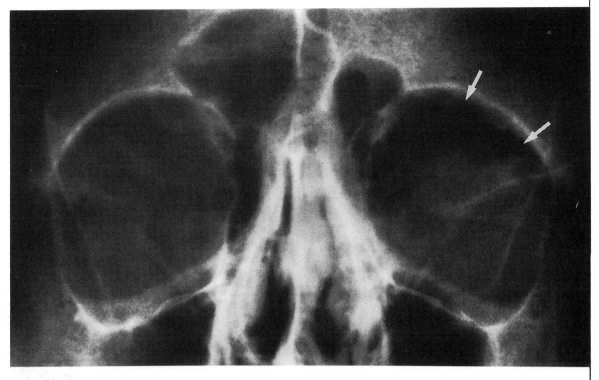

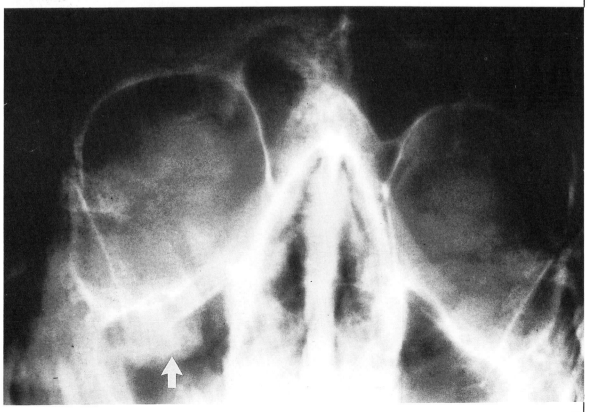

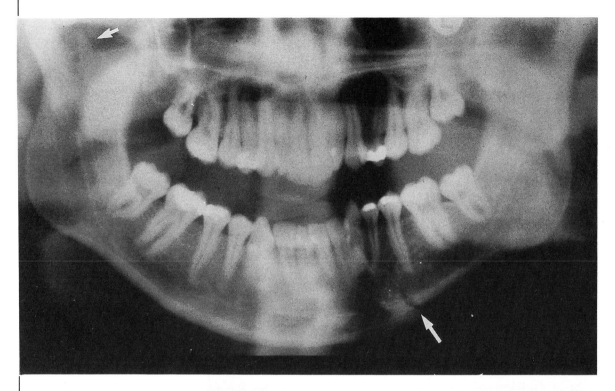

Figure 1.13. (Above). Orthopantomogram of the mandible. There is a fracture of the left side of the body of the mandible and also of the neck of the right condyle.

Figure 1.14. (Right). Anteroposterior view of the mandible of Figure 1.13 showing the condylar neck fracture more clearly.

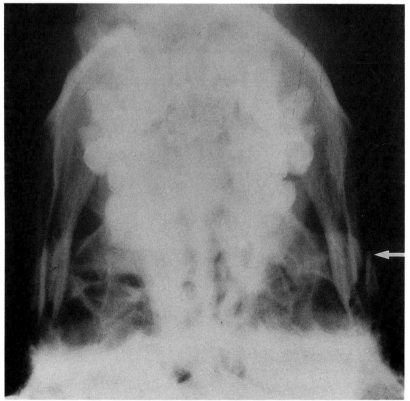

● BIBLIOGRAPHY ●

Alley, R. H. (1964) Head and neck injuries in high school football. *J. Am. Med. Ass.* **118**, 118.

American Medical Association, Council on Scientific Affairs (1983) Brain injury in boxing. *J. Am. Med. Ass.* **249**, 254.

Avery, J. G. (1988) Sporting motorcycle accidents in children. *Public Health* **102(1)**, 27.

Barth, J. T., Macciocchi, S. N., Giordani, B., Rimel, R., Jane, J. A. and Boll, T. J. (1983) Neuro-psychological sequelae of minor head injury. *Neurosurgery* **13(5)**, 529.

Belongia, E., et al. (1988) Severity and types of head trauma among adult bicycle riders. *Wis. Med. J.* **87(1)**, 11.

Bogholi, L. R., et al. (1987) Harness racing injuries and deaths. *Am. J. For. Med. Pathol.* **8**, 185.

Bolhuis, J. H. A., Leurs, J. M. M. and Plogel, G. E. (1987) Dental and facial injuries in international field hockey. *Brit. J. Sports Med.* **21(4)**, 174.

Brennan, T. N. and O'Connor, P. J. (1968) Incidence of boxing injuries in the Royal Air Force in the United Kingdom 1953-66. *Br. J. Industr. Med.* **25**, 326.

British Medical Association (1984) Boxing: Report of the Board of Science and Education Working Party.

Bruno, L. A. (1982) Focal intracranial hematoma. In: Torg, J. S. (ed.) *Athletic Injuries to the Head, Neck and Face.* Philadelphia: Lea & Febiger.

Buckley, W. E. (1988) Concussions in college football. A multivariate analysis. *Am. J. Sports Med.* **16(1)**, 51.

Casson, I., Shaw, R. and Campbell, E. (1982) The neurological and CT evaluation of the knocked-out boxer. *J. Neurol. Neurosurg. Psych.* **45**, 170.

Casson, I., Siegel, O., Shaw R., et al. (1984) Brain damage in modern boxing. *J. Am. Med. Ass.* **250**, 2663.

Corsellis, J., Bruton, C. and Freeman-Browne, D. (1983) The aftermath of boxing. *Psychol. Med.* **3**, 270.

Critchley, M. (1957) Medical aspects of boxing, particularly from the neurological standpoint. *Br. Med. J.* **1**, 357.

Cruikshank, J. K., Higgens, C. S. and Gray, J. R. (1980) Two cases of intracranial haemorrhage in young amateur boxers. *Lancet* **i**, 626.

Danielsson, L. G. and Westlin, N. E. (1973) Riding accidents. *Acta Orthop. Scand.* **44**, 497.

East, C. A., et al. (1987) Acute nasal trauma in children. *J. Pediatr. Surg.* **22**, 308.

Enzenauer, R. W., et al. (1987) Ban military boxing. *Milit. Med.* **152**, 637.

Feriencik, K. (1979) Case report: depressed skull fracture in an ice hockey player wearing a helmet. *Phys. Sports Med.* **7**, 107.

Fischer, C. M. (1966) Concussion amnesia. *Neurology* **16**, 826.

Garon, W. M., Merkle, A. and Wright, J. T. (1986) Mouth protectors and oral trauma: a study of adolescent football players. *J. Am. Dent. Ass.* **112**, 663.

Gierup, J., Larsson, M. and Lennquist, S. (1976) Incidence and nature of horse riding injuries. *Acta Chir. Scand.* **142**, 57.

Han, J. S., Kaufman, B., Alfidi, R. J., et al. (1984) Head trauma evaluated by magnetic resonance and computed tomography: a comparison. *Neuroradiology* **150(1)**, 71.

Jones, N. P., et al. (1986) Severe eye injuries in cricket. *Br. J. Sports Med.* **20**, 178.

Jones, N. P. (1987) Eye injuries in sport: an increasing problem. *Brit. J. Sports Med.* **21**, 168.

Jordan, B. D. (1987) Neurologic aspects of boxing. *Arch. Neurol.* **44**, 453.

Kelly, S. P. (1987) Serious eye injury in badminton players. *Br. J. Ophthalmology* **71**, 746.

Lampert, P. W. and Hardman, J. M. (1984) Morphologic changes in brains of boxers. *J. Am. Med. Ass.* **251**, 2676.

Landsman, I. S., Knapp, J. F., Medina, F., Sharma, V., Wasserman, G. S., and Walsh, I. (1987) Injuries associated with downhill sledding. *Paed. Emerg. Care* **3(4)**, 277.

Lehman, L. B. (1987) Sports related CNS injuries in children and adolescents. *Postgrad. Med.* **82**, 141.

McEwen, C. J. (1987) Sport associated eye injuries. *Br. J. Ophthalmology* **71**, 701.

McLatchie, G. R., Davies, J. E. and Gaulley, J. H. (1980) Injuries in karate. *J. Trauma* **20**, 956.

McLatchie, G., et al. (1987) Clinical neurological examination, neuro-psychology, electro-encephalography and computed tomography in active amateur boxers. *J. Neurol. Neurosurg. Psych.* **50**, 96.

Matthews, W. B. N. (1972) Footballers' migraine. *Br. Med. J.* **2**, 326.

Mawdsley, C. and Ferguson, F. R. (1983) Neurological disease in boxers. *Lancet* **ii**, 795.

Morrow, P. L., McQuillen, E. N., Eaton, L. A. and Bernstein, C. J. (1988) Downhill ski fatalities: the Vermont experience. *J. Trauma* **28**, 95.

Myers, P. T. (1980) Injuries presenting from Rugby Union Football. *Med. J. Aust.* **2**, 17.

Nysether, S. (1987) Dental injuries amongst Norwegian soccer players. *Community Dent. Oral Epidemiol.* **15**, 141.

Pashby, T. (1987) Eye injuries in Canadian amateur hockey, still a concern. *Can. J. Ophthalmol.* **22(6)**, 293.

Ross, R. J., Cole, M., Thompson, J. S. and Kim, K. H. (1983) Boxers: computed tomography, E. E. G. and neurological evaluation. *J. Am. Med. Ass.* **249**, 211.

Royal College of Physicians of London (1969) Committee on Boxing: Report on the medical aspects of boxing.

Ryan, A. J. (1979) A hit in the head. *Physician and Sports Med.* **7**, 49.

Sabharwal, R. K., *et al.* (1987) Chronic traumatic encephalopathy in boxers. *J. Ass. Phys. India* **35(8)**, 571.

Sane, J., *et al.* (1987) Maxillofacial and dental soccer injuries in Finland. *Br. J. Oral Maxillofac. Surg.* **25**, 383.

Schneider, R. C. (1966) Serious and fatal neurosurgical football injuries. *Clin. Neurosurg.* **12**, 236.

Siana, J. E., Borum, P. and Kryger, H. (1986) Injuries in Taekwondo. *Br. J. Sports Med.* **20**, 165.

Spillane, J. D. (1962) Five boxers. *Br. Med. J.* **2**, 1205.

Tysvaer, A. and Storli, O. (1981) Association football injuries to the brain. A preliminary report. *Br. J. Sports Med.* **15**, 163.

Worrell, J. (1987) Head injuries in pedal cyclists. *Injury* **18(1)**, 5.

Wright, J. R. (1988) Nordic ski jumping fatalities in the United States. A 50-year summary. *J. Trauma* **28(6)**, 848.

Yarnell, P. R. and Lynch, S. (1973) The "ding": amnestic states in football trauma. *Neurology* **23**, 186.

2 The Cervical Spine

Minor injuries to the neck are seen frequently in any sports medicine practice and occur in a wide variety of athletic pursuits. More significant damage, such as fractures and fracture/dislocations to the region, is fortunately a less common occurrence. The major problem with these more serious injuries is the involvement of the cervical cord with the catastrophic sequelae which then ensue.

The brute sports such as gridiron football, rugby and wrestling are obviously activities that can lead to cervical spine damage, but sports such as diving, gymnastics, skiing and ice hockey all produce a small but significant number of bad neck injuries. Further, the cumulative effect of many minor injuries to the area also produces long-term structural damage which can lead to significant symptoms developing late in the athlete's career or even after retirement. The commonest mechanism producing injuries to the neck in sport is hyperflexion, although hyperextension injuries do occasionally occur particularly in activities such as gymnastics.

In the period immediately following a neck injury where there has been damage to an intervertebral disc, no changes would be visible on a plain radiograph. An MRI scan, however, as in the young man with an acutely injured neck shown in Figure 2.1, may demonstrate the ruptured herniated disc, probably even before the problem is seen on a myelogram or CT myelogram.

Subsequently changes appear such as the disc space narrowing shown in Figure 2.2 which is a lateral view of the cervical spine of a 29-year-old rugby player who damaged his neck in a 'head-on' tackle two years before this film was taken. In American football the tackling technique known as 'spearing' produces cervical spine injuries by the same mechanism, *i.e.* a heavy direct blow on the vertex produces a high axial loading on the cervical vertebrae. Figure 2.2 also shows a narrowed cervical canal, particularly in the C4–C5 region where the ratio of the diameter of the canal to the vertebral body is less than one. This abnormality sometimes gives rise to an acute, but transient, neuropraxia originating from the cervical cord immediately after an injury; this player experienced a severe burning pain in his arms and hands and a period of weakness in his right forearm and hand, following a torsion injury to his neck in a scrum.

Later, bony changes such as large osteophytes can develop at the site of injury, as shown in the view of the neck of the 35-year-old rugby player which is reproduced in Figure 2.3. This was consequent upon an injury sustained some ten years previously, and on occasions this type of damage can proceed to bony ankylosis.

Injuries to supporting structures such as the interspinous ligaments and the anterior and posterior longitudinal ligaments, as with intervertebral disc injuries, are not in themselves visible on conventional radiographs. The presence of an anterior spinal haematoma (see Figure 2.18) on a plain film may give an indication that such an injury has occurred, while a detectable widening of the interspinous gap (*i.e.* the gap between two successive spinous processes) found on clinical

Figure 2.1. (Below left). MRI scan of a young man demonstrating a ruptured annulus with herniation of the nucleus pulposus.

Figure 2.2. (Below right). Lateral view of the cervical spine showing a narrowed C5–C6 disc (arrow) following a previously documented injury.

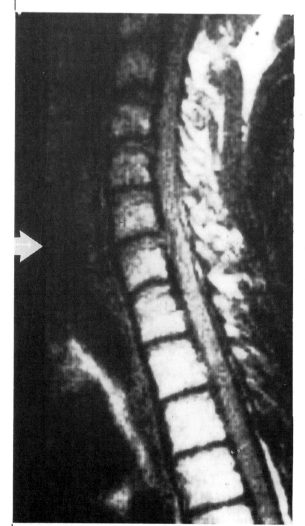

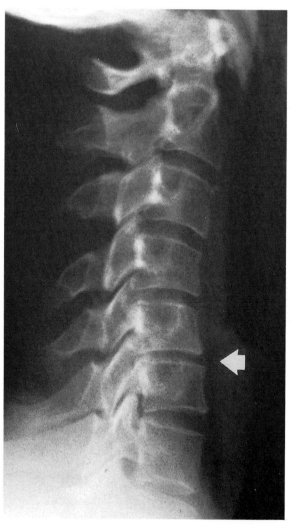

12

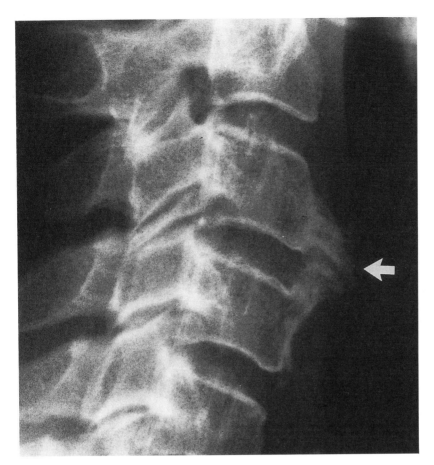

Figure 2.3. Localized view of C3–C4 showing gross osteophyte formation in a rugby player, secondary to an injury some ten years previously.

examination is of great significance. Figure 2.4 is a lateral view of the cervical spine of a 25-year-old man which shows slightly abnormal angulation between the third and fourth cervical vertebrae with co-existing widening of the interspinous gap. This is an unstable injury and its significance was not appreciated by the junior doctor who reviewed the film; a further minor injury subsequently resulted in the C3–C4 subluxation shown in Figure 2.5. Fortunately there were no permanent neurological sequelae and internal fixation was undertaken with good results.

Fractures of the spinous processes of the cervical vertebrae, usually the lower ones, occur secondary to muscular action in the so-called 'clay shoveller's' injury. We have however, occasionally seen this type of damage in the contact sports as in Figure 2.6 which demonstrates a fracture to the spinous process of C4 in a 21-year-old judo black belt. Classically the 'clay shoveller's' fracture is a stable one; however, this particular injury extended into the laminae and thus is potentially unstable. Such patients should be kept under review as there may be a gradual progression to a flexion deformity over the following 12 months or so.

Violent hyperflexion or hyperextension injuries to the neck may

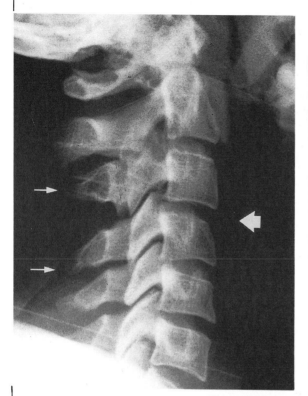

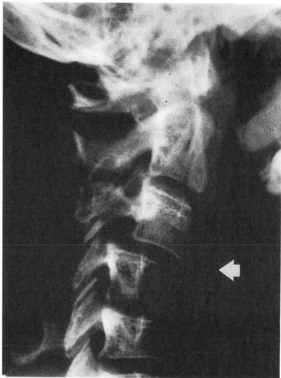

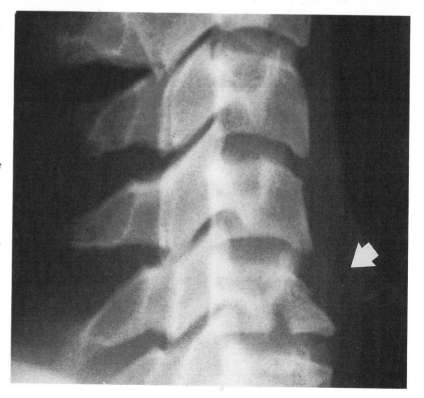

Figure 2.4. (Above left). Lateral cervical spine film of a young man showing slightly abnormal angulation anteriorly between C3 and C4, together with widening of the interspinous gap at this level indicating that this is an unstable injury with ruptured ligaments.

Figure 2.5. (Above right.) Same patient as Figure 2.4 but following a further minor injury. This shows a subluxation of C3 on C4.

Figure 2.6. (Right). Fracture of the spinous process of C4. This is not a simple 'clay shoveller's' injury as it extends into the laminae and is potentially unstable.

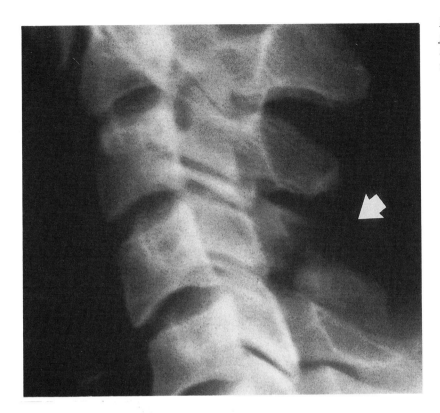

Figure 2.7. Classical 'tear-drop' fracture of the body of C5 due to a violent hyperextension injury.

produce fractures of the vertebral bodies without injury to the spinal cord. These lesions are usually stable, although where there are associated neurological abnormalities further investigation, preferably with MRI or CT, is necessary. Figure 2.7 illustrates a 'tear-drop' fracture of the body of C5 caused by the violent hyperextension of the neck produced by a 'stiff arm' tackle in a 24-year-old man.

A facet fracture can be difficult to pick up although careful screening using fluoroscopy and image intensification may help to demonstrate it; further minor degrees of instability can also be detected using these techniques. Facet dislocations can also be hard to visualize on conventional films and again may require further exhaustive investigations using other techniques. Where clinical suspicions exist in patients who have sustained a significant neck injury but have apparently normal routine films, further investigation should be undertaken to look for more subtle problems. One such is illustrated in Figure 2.8 in the neck of a 20-year-old gymnast who has a unifacet dislocation at the C3-C4 level.

Fractures in the upper part of the neck usually involve the neural arch of C2, producing the so-called 'hangman's' fractures that result from hyperextension injuries, as was the one illustrated in Figures 2.9 and 2.10. If the hyperextension is associated with distraction then death results as in judicial hanging. Such injuries have occurred in accidents involving certain all-terrain vehicles such as snowmobiles.

Another injury that occurs high in the cervical spine is disruption of the bony ring of C1, the so-called 'Jefferson' fracture which is the equivalent of a burst fracture of one of the other cervical vertebral bodies. It occurs where a diver lands on the vertex of the skull and the occipital condyles impinge forcibly on the atlas, bursting open the ring. This was the mechanism in the case illustrated in Figure 2.12 (Figure 2.11 is a normal for comparison). These fractures are easily missed if not specifically looked for, although fortunately, as with the more common fractures of the odontoid peg, the patients are usually neurologically intact.

When neck injuries occur in older individuals they sometimes appear to be complicated by problems with the vascular supply to the spinal

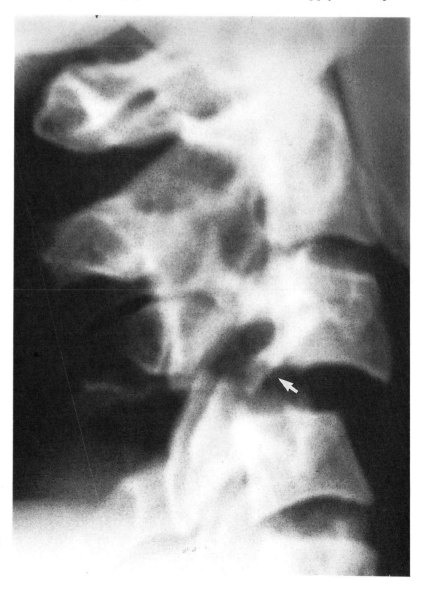

Figure 2.8. Unifacet dislocation at the C3–C4 level. The dislocated facet is arrowed.

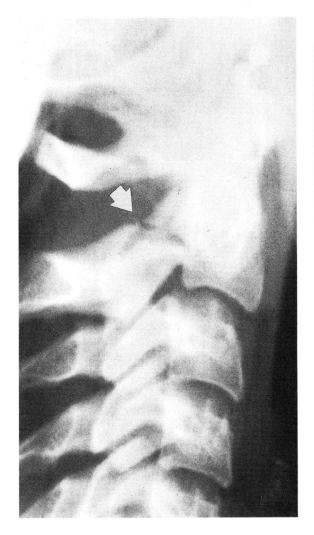
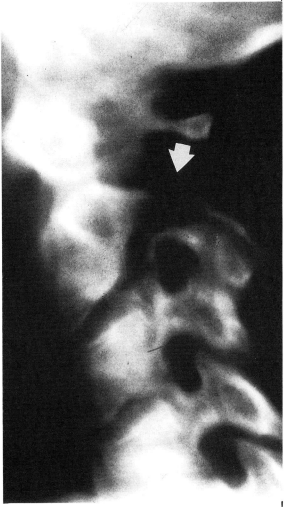

cord. Significant neurological signs and symptoms can be present in the absence of any detectable bony injury. Even at surgery no abnormality may be found, and further, long-standing degenerative changes that may be seen on plain radiographs can mislead as in the case illustrated in Figures 2.13 and 2.14. The original film (Figure 2.13) was taken when a 46-year-old man was seen following an injury to his neck sustained while playing five-a-side soccer indoors in a gymnasium. This X-ray was thought to show only spondylotic changes that were obviously long-standing, but no recent injury, and even on retrospective viewing no abnormality could be definitely identified. One week later a follow-up X-ray (Figure 2.14) clearly revealed that the patient was developing a marked angular kyphosis at C5–C6; the interspinous gap was wide, and C5 had displaced forward on C6 indicating that the patient must have disrupted the interspinous and longitudinal ligaments in the course of the original injury. We feel that in such patients due

Figure 2.9. (Above left). 'Hangman's' fracture of C2 due to a hyperextension injury.

Figure 2.10. (Above right). 'Hangman's' fracture more clearly demonstrated by the use of tomography.

consideration should be given to screening the cervical spine by a senior radiologist, otherwise instability can be readily overlooked.

Further we should stress that no X-ray examination of the neck is complete without demonstrating the full length of the cervical spine down to and including the seventh cervical vertebra. This can often be difficult, particularly in people with a short muscular neck, so if necessary the patient should be screened using fluoroscopy, or have tomography performed. Figure 2.15 shows a coned view of the lower cervical spine in a young girl who was tetraplegic following a diving accident. The initial films had shown no apparent abnormality but C7 had not been demonstrated, and further views clearly illustrated a burst fracture of the body of that vertebra. This finding was confirmed by a CT scan which did not, however, show any bony fragments within the spinal canal (Figure 2.16).

CT scanning, particularly when combined with the injection of contrast medium into the thecal sac, can demonstrate the anatomy of the cervical spine quite elegantly. However, in selected cases MRI should be performed as it is the only technique that can demonstrate the bones, soft tissue anatomy and the substance of the spinal cord. This is well illustrated in Figures 2.17 and 2.18, where the original plain films (Figure 2.17) taken shortly after the injury raised suspicions of a fracture of the odontoid peg, although the patient's neurological signs had been thought to have been secondary to a central cord lesion due to vascular damage. An MRI scan (Figure 2.18) confirmed the presence of a fracture through the base of the odontoid with a collection of blood (a prevertebral haematoma) lying anterior to the upper cervical spine. There was also damage to the spinal cord visible at the level of C2, although no significant abnormality lower in the cervical spine could be seen. The odontoid peg subsequently united satisfactorily and the patient made a good recovery.

Figure 2.11. Open-mouth view of the odontoid peg showing the normal relationship of C1 facets on C2.

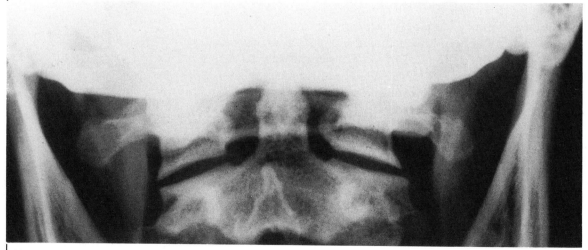

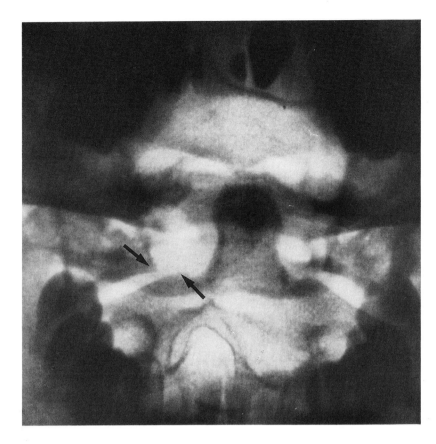

Figure 2.12. (Left). Open-mouth view of the odontoid showing displacement of the facets of C1 on C2 due to a 'Jefferson' fracture of the neural arch of C1.

Figure 2.13. (Below left). Lateral of the cervical spine of a 46-year-old man showing spondylotic changes at C5–C6 and C6–C7 but otherwise normal.

Figure 2.14. (Below right). Follow-up X-ray of same patient as Figure 2.13 taken one week later showing a progressive flexion deformity at C5–C6 due to disruption of the interspinous ligament and the disc.

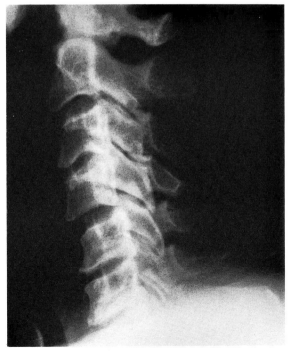

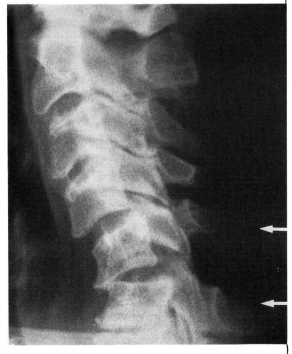

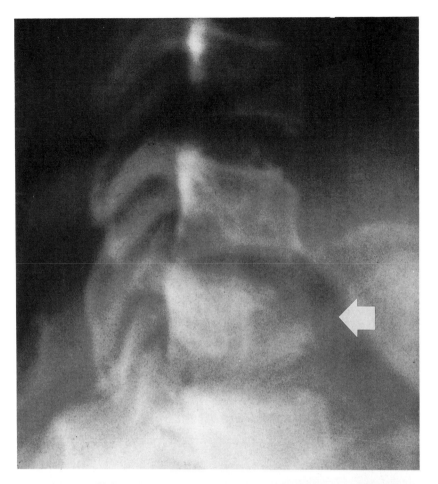

Figure 2.15. Fracture of the body of C7 in a young girl following a diving accident.

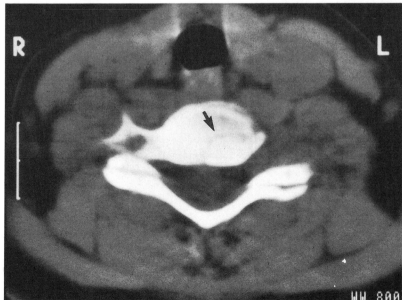

Figure 2.16. CT scan of the same case as in Figure 2.15 showing a fracture of the body of C7 but no bony fragments in the spinal canal.

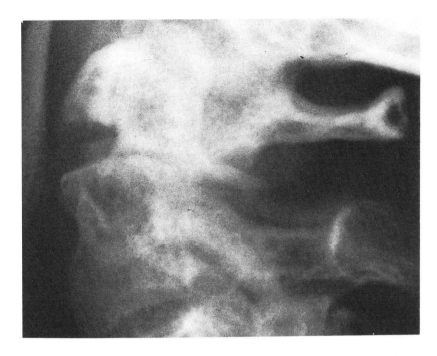

Figure. 2.17. Coned lateral view of the cervical spine showing a suspicious appearance of the odontoid peg, possibly projectional.

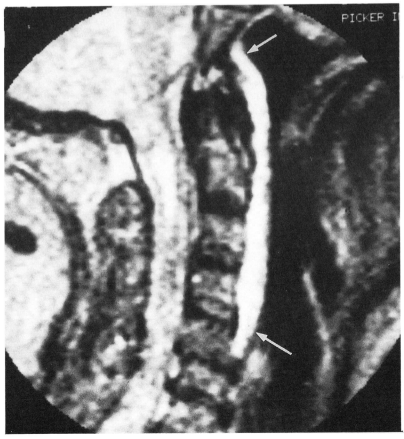

Figure 2.18. MRI scan of the case shown in Figure 2.17, clearly demonstrating the presence of blood anterior to the upper cervical spine, fracture of the odontoid peg, and haemorrhage in the spinal cord at C2 level.

• BIBLIOGRAPHY •

Albrand, O. W. and Walter, J. (1975) Underwater deceleration curves in relation to injuries from diving. *Surg. Neurol.* **4**, 461.

Beatson, T. R. (1963) Fractures and dislocations of the cervical spine. *J. Bone Joint Surg.* **45(B)**, 21.

Binet, E. F., Moro, J. J., Marnagola, J. P., *et al.* (1977) Cervical spine tomography in trauma. *Spine* **2**, 163.

Brown, B. M., *et al.* (1982) Dynamic CT scanning of spinal column trauma. *Am. J. Radiol.* **139**, 1177.

Burry, H. C. and Calcinai, C. J. (1988) The need to make rugby safer. *Br. Med. J.* **296**, 149.

Clarke, K. W. (1977) A survey of sports-related spinal cord injuries in schools and colleges, 1973–1975. *J. Safety Res.* **9**, 140.

Coin, C. G., Pennick, M., Ahmad, W. D. and Keranen, V. J. (1979) Diving-type injury to the cervical spine: contribution of computed tomography to management. *J. Comput. Assist. Tomogr.* **3(3)**, 362.

Enzmann, D. R. and Rubin, J. B. (1988) Cervical spine: M. R. Imaging with a partial flip angle. *Radiology* **166**, 467.

Epstein, V. A., Epstein, J. A. and Jones, M. D. (1977) Cervical spinal stenosis. *Radiol. Clin. North Am.* **15**, 215.

Evans, D. K. (1976) Anterior cervical subluxation. *J. Bone Joint Surg.* **55(B)**, 318.

Evans, R. F. (1979) Tetraplegia caused by gymnastics. *Br. Med. J.* **2**, 732.

Frostik, S. P., Catterson, J. and Duthie, R. B. (1986) Spinal injuries to young rugby players in the Oxford region. *Health Trends* **18**, 43.

Gerlock, A. J. Jr. and Mirfakhraee, M. (1983) CT and Hangman's fractures. *South Med. J.* **76**, 727.

Govender, S. and Charles, R. W. (1987) Traumatic spondylolisthesis of the axis. *Injury* **18**, 333.

Hitchcock, E. R. and Karmi, M. A. (1982) Sports injuries to the cervical spinal cord. *J. R. Coll. Surg.* **27**, 46.

Horan, F. T. (1984) Injuries to the cervical spine in schoolboys playing rugby football. *J. Bone Joint Surg.* **66(B)**, 470.

Jefferson, G. (1920) Fracture of the atlas vertebra. *Br. J. Surg.* **7**, 407.

Kessler, J. T. (1975) Congenital narrowing of the cervical spinal canal. *J. Neurol. Neurosurg. Psych.* **38**, 1218.

Kewalramani, L. S. and Kraus, J. F. (1981) Cervical spine injuries resulting from collision sports. *Paraplegia* **19**, 303.

Kewalramani, L. S. and Thomas, R. G. (1975) Injuries to the cervical spine from diving accidents. *J. Trauma* **15**, 130.

Kulkarni, M. V., McArdle, C. B., Kopanicky, D., *et al.* (1987) Acute spinal cord injury. M.R. Imaging at 1.5T. *Radiology* **164**, 837.

Kurtzke, J. F. (1975) Epidemiology of spinal cord injury. *Exp. Neurol.* **48**, 163.

Leidholt, D. J. (1963) Spinal injury in sports. *Surg. Clin. North Am.* **143**, 351.

Mace, S. E. (1985) Emergency evaluation of cervical spine injuries: C.T. versus plain radiographs. *Ann. Emerg. Med.* **14**, 973.

McPhee, I. B. (1981) Spinal fractures and dislocations in children and adolescents. *Spine* **6**, 533.

Mirvis, S. E., *et al.* (1987) Hangman's fracture: radiologic assessment in 37 cases. *Radiology* **163**, 714.

Morrow, P. L., McQuillen, E. N., Eaton, L. A. and Bernstein, C. J. (1988) Downhill ski fatalities: the Vermont experience. *J. Trauma* **28**, 95.

O'Brien, P. J., Schweigel, J. F. and Thompson, W. J. (1983) Dislocations of the lower cervical spine. *J. Trauma* **22**, 710.

O'Carroll, P. F., Gregg, T. M. and Sheehan, J. M. (1981) Cervical spine injuries in rugby football. *Irish Med. J.* **74**, 12.

Oh, S. (1984) Cervical injuries from skiing. *Int. J. Sports Med.* **5**, 268.

Pavlov, H., Torg, J. S., Robe, B. and Jahre, C. (1987) Cervical spine stenosis: determination with vertebral body ratio method. *Radiology* **164**, 771.

Penning, L. (1981) Prevertebral haematoma in cervical spine injury: incidence and etiological significance. *Am. J. Radiol.* **136**, 553.

Post, M. J. F., *et al.* (1982) The value of computed tomography in spinal trauma. *Spine* **7**, 417.

Rapp, G. F. and Nicely, P. G. (1978) Trampoline injuries. *Am. J. Sports Med.* **6**, 269.

Reid, D. C., Henderson, R., Soboe, L. and Miller, J. D. R. (1987) Etiology and clinical course of missed spine fractures. *J. Trauma* **27**, 980.

Scher, A. T. (1978) The high rugby tackle—an avoidable cause of cervical spinal cord injury. *S. Afr. Med. J.* **53**, 1015.

Scher, A. T. (1980) The value of retropharyngeal swelling in the diagnosis of fractures of the atlas. *S. Afr. Med. J.* **58**, 451.

Scher, A. T. (1987) Rugby injuries of the spine and spinal cord. *Clin. Sports Med.* **6**, 87.

Shields, C. L. Jr., Fox, J. M. and Stauffer, E. S. (1978) Cervical cord injuries in sports. *Phys. Sportsmed.* **6**, 71.

Silver, J. R. (1984) Injuries of the spine sustained in rugby. *Br. Med. J.* **288**, 37.

Stauffer, E. S. and Kelly, E. G. (1977) Fracture-dislocations of the cervical spine. *J. Bone Joint Surg.* **59(A)**, 45.

Tarr, R. W., Drolshagen, L. F., Kerner, T. C., *et al.* (1987) M.R. Imaging of recent spinal trauma. *J. Comput. Assist. Tomogr.* **11**, 412.

Tator, C. H. (1987) Neck injuries in ice hockey. *Clin. Sports Med.* **6**, 101.

Tator, C. H. and Edmonds, V. E. (1984) National survey of spinal injuries in hockey players. *Can. Med. Ass. J.* **130**, 875.

Tator, C. H., Edmonds, V. E. and New, M. L. (1981) Diving: a frequent and potentially preventable cause of spinal cord injury. *Can. Med. Ass. J.* **124**, 1323.

Taylor, T. K. F. and Coolican, M. R. J. (1987) Spinal cord injuries in Australian footballers. 1960-1985. *Med. J. Aust.* **147**, 112.

Torg, J. S. (1985) Epidemiology, pathomechanics, and prevention of athletic injuries to the cervical spine. *Med. Sci. Sports Exerc.* **7**, 295.

Torg, J. S. (1987) Trampoline-induced quadriplegia. *Clin. Sports Med.* **6**, 73.

Torg, J. S. and Pavlov, H. (1987) Cervical spinal stenosis with cord neuropraxia and transient quadriplegia. *Clin. Sports Med.* **6**, 115.

Torg, J. S., Vegso, J. J., Sennett, B. and Das, M. (1985) The national football head and neck injury registry. 14-year report on cervical quadriplegia, 1971 through 1984. *J. Am. Med. Ass.* **254**, 3439.

Weir, D. C. (1975) Roentgenographic signs of cervical injury. *Clin. Orthop.* **109**, 9.

Williams, J. P. and McKibbin, B. (1987) Unstable cervical spine injuries in rugby—a 20 year review. *Injury* **18**, 329.

3 The Chest

Minor injuries to the chest and pectoral muscles are common in many sporting activities and are rarely worthy of radiological investigation. The commonest bony injury in our experience is a rib fracture, usually the middle ribs on the lateral aspect of the chest wall. As long as there has been no damage to the underlying lung, resolution is normally satisfactory although a painful process. Damage to the costochondral junction in contact sports is also seen quite frequently but here radiographs are unhelpful. To demonstrate rib fractures adequately, oblique views are often necessary (Figure 3.1) as in this 22-year-old wrestler. Normal posteroanterior chest films in inspiration and expiration will exclude a pneumothorax but fractures to the ribs may be missed due to the curvature of the bones.

Injuries to the clavicle are most frequent at its acromial end and to the mid-shaft, but problems do occur at the sternoclavicular junction and these can be difficult to demonstrate radiologically, although clinically the diagnosis is usually obvious. Anterior subluxation/ dislocation is the most common problem at this joint and is best demonstrated by CT scanning, as is the rarer and far more serious posterior dislocation.

Tomograms as illustrated in Figure 3.2 can also delineate the lesion. Tomography is the investigation that is most commonly available in radiology departments. The film shown here was obtained on a young rugby player.

As with other bones the ribs are subject to stress fractures, although these are uncommon. The most widely recognized is the lesion to the first rib and this has been described in hikers/back-packers, weight-lifters, *etc*. Figure 3.3 is the chest X-ray of a 32-year-old man who had covered a distance of some 11 miles carrying his pack when he began to experience persistent pain at the base of the neck anteriorly; over the previous month he had averaged 35 miles per week, usually with a pack. His chest X-rays revealed abnormal first ribs and a more localized view (Figure 3.4) confirmed the presence of bilateral stress fractures.

Care should be taken when interpreting abnormalities in this area as it is not uncommon to have cervical ribs with extra joints or fragments of bones at their ends. If there is serious doubt about the clinical diagnosis, bone scanning with isotopes is useful to differentiate between a true fracture and a normal variant.

Injuries to the sternum are uncommon and are caused only by significant violence as, for instance, in accidents in sports such as parachuting, hang-gliding, skiing and incidents involving all-terrain vehicles, as in Figure 3.5. Either the manubrium or the body of the sternum may be involved, with or without displacement, and the presence of a retrosternal haematoma may give a clue to the diagnosis on plain films. While direct blows to the sternum can result in a simple sternal fracture as shown in Figure 3.5, one should always be aware of the association between sternal fractures and fractures of the thoracic spine. These injuries are usually caused by sudden violent flexion, and Figure 3.6 demonstrates a fracture of the body of the sternum together with a compression fracture of the body of one of the thoracic vertebrae. These spinal lesions may be unstable when accompanied by sternal and rib fractures, and where this is the case the patient is at serious risk of neurological damage. If the thoracic spine does deform there is almost invariably injury to the thoracic cord as the canal has little spare capacity

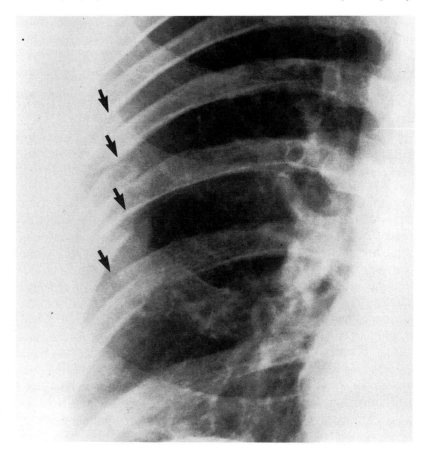

Figure 3.1. Oblique view of the chest demonstrating multiple rib fractures.

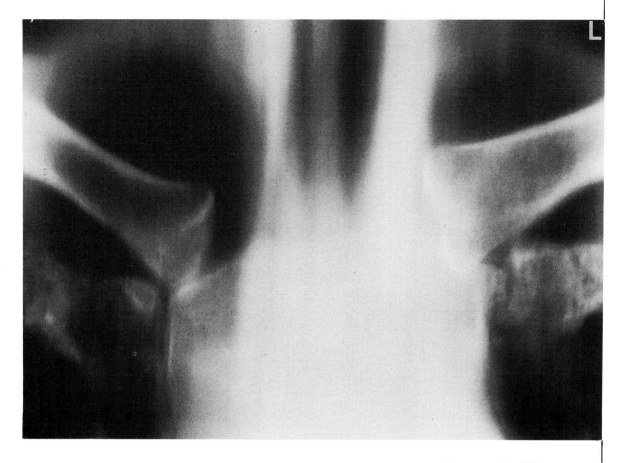

L

Figure 3.2. Magnified tomographic view of the sternoclavicular joints. The left is subluxated with displacement of the clavicle superiorly and anteriorly.

in this region. The results are usually catastrophic as can be seen from the case illustrated in Figure 3.7 which is an MRI film showing a fracture of the vertebral body with angulation and some displacement.

Intrathoracic structures may also be damaged in this type of incident and if there has been a major deceleration element the aorta may be transected. Where this diagnosis is a serious possibility, either angiography, CT or MRI should be undertaken as an urgent diagnostic procedure.

Highly trained athletes develop a cardiomegaly and a bradycardia. Figure 3.8 is the posteroanterior chest film of a 25-year-old international class marathon/cross-country runner who had a heart rate of 48 per minute. As well as the marked bradycardia, the electrocardiogram may show other 'abnormalities' which, in association with the cardiomegaly seen on a plain PA chest film, can give rise to mistaken diagnoses of cardiac disease. Unfortunately, however, there is well documented evidence of sudden death occurring in young athletes who were previously regarded as fit. Death is usually due to an unrecognized cardiomyopathy or to ischaemic heart disease. In view of these circumstances, complaints by athletes of chest pain or palpitations should never be ignored.

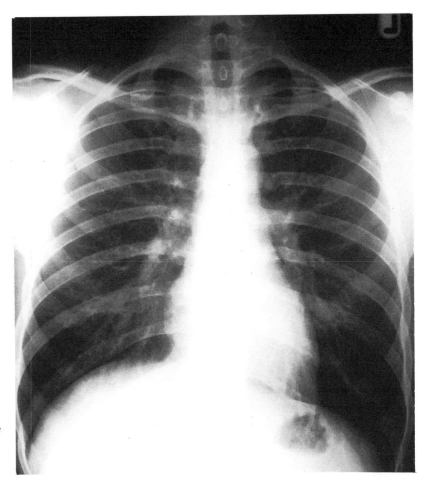

Figure 3.3. (Right). Posteroanterior chest X-ray. The appearances of the first ribs are suspicious, otherwise the chest is normal.

Figure 3.4. (Below). Localized view of the first ribs (same case as in Figure 3.3) confirming an abnormality due to a bilateral pseudoarthrosis.

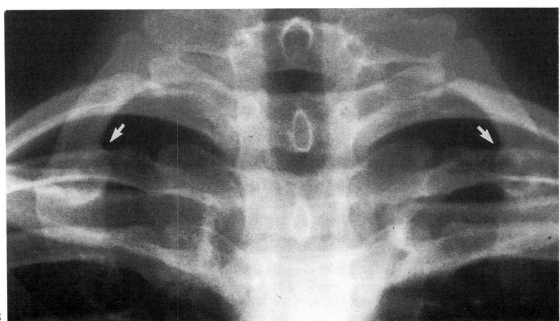

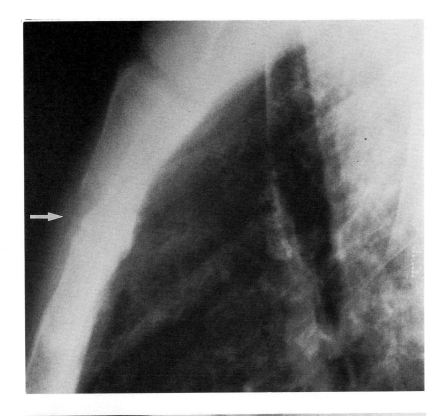

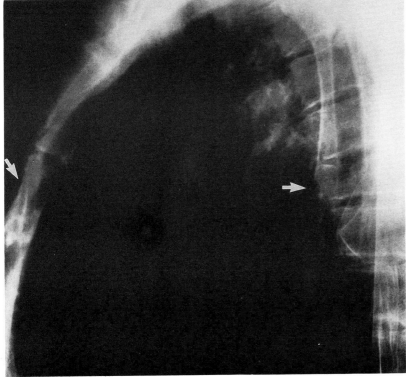

Figure 3.5. (Above). Lateral X-ray of the sternum demonstrating a displaced fracture of the manubrium.

Figure 3.6. (Left). Over-penetrated lateral chest X-ray. There is a displaced fracture of the sternum and an associated fracture of one of the thoracic vertebral bodies.

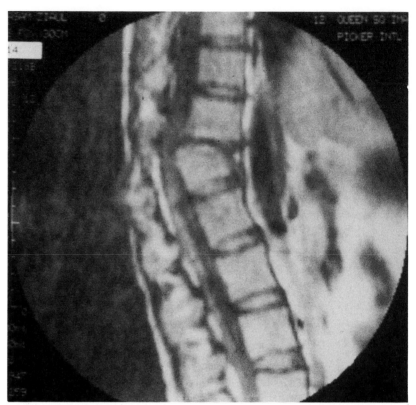

Figure 3.7. MRI scan of the thoracic spine showing a fracture of the vertebral body with angulation and some displacement. The posterior displacement is compressing the spinal cord.

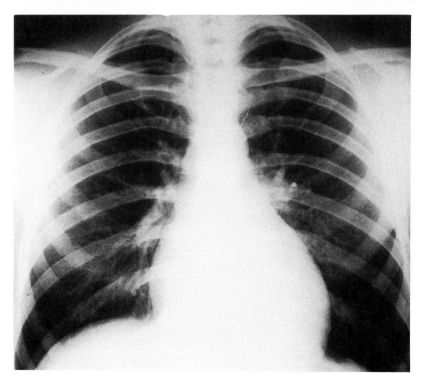

Figure 3.8. Posteroanterior chest X-ray in a young adult male showing a moderately enlarged heart secondary to his athletic activity.

● BIBLIOGRAPHY ●

Barber, H. M. (1973) Horse-play: survey of accidents with horses. *Br. Med. J.* **3**, 532.

DeLuca, S. A., Rhea, J. T. and O'Malley, T. (1982) Radiographic evaluation of rib fractures. *Am. J. Radiol.* **138**, 91.

Destouet, J. M., Gilula, L. A., Murphy, W. A., *et al.* (1981) Computed tomography of the sternoclavicular joint and sternum. *Radiology* **138**, 123.

Devas, M. D. (1979) Stress fractures of the ribs. *Proc. R. Soc. Med.* **62**, 936.

Ekblom, B. and Hermansen, L. (1968) Cardiac outputs in athletes. *J. Appl. Physiol.* **25**, 619.

Evans, R. (1980) Sudden death in sportsmen. *Medisport* **2**, 298.

Fam, A. G. and Smythe, H. A. (1985) Musculoskeletal chest wall pain. *Can. Med. Ass. J.* **133**, 379.

Fowler, A. W. (1957) Flexion–compression injury of the sternum. *J. Bone Joint Surg.* **39(B)**, 487.

Freiberger, R. H. and Mayer, V. (1964) Ununited bilateral fractures of the 1st ribs. *J. Bone Joint Surg.* **46(A)**, 615.

Gopalkrishnan, K. C. and El Masri, W. S. (1986) Fractures of the sternum associated with spinal injury. *J. Bone Joint Surg.* **68(B)**, 178.

Gurtler, R. (1985) Stress fracture of the ipsilateral first rib in a pitcher. *Am. J. Sports Med.* **13**, 277.

Hanne-Papafo, N., Drory, Y., Schoenfeld, Y., *et al.* (1976) Common E.C.G. changes in athletes. *Cardiology* **61**, 267.

Harkonen, M., *et al.* (1969) Fractures of the thoracic spine. *Arch. Orthop. Traum. Surg.* **94**, 179.

Holden, D. and Jackson, D. (1985) Stress fracture of the ribs in female rowers. *Am. J. Sports Med.* **13**, 342.

Kilcoyne, R. F., Mack, L. A., King, H. A., *et al.* (1983) Thoracolumbar spine injuries associated with vertical plunges: reappraisal with computed tomography. *Radiology* **146**, 137.

Levinsohn, E. M., Bunell, W. and Yuan, H. (1979) Computed tomography in the diagnosis of dislocations of the sternoclavicular joint. *Clin. Orthop.* **140**, 12.

Lichtman, J., O'Rourke, R. A., Klein, A., *et al.* (1973) Electrocardiogram of the athlete. Alternations simulating those of organic heart disease. *Arch. Intern. Med.* **132**, 763.

Malcolm, B. M. (1979) Pneumothorax complicating a fracture of the clavicle. *Can. J. Surg.* **22**, 84.

Maron, B. J., Roberts, W. C., McAlister, H. A., *et al.* (1980) Sudden death in young athletes. *Circulation* **62(2)**, 218.

Morganroth, J., Maron, B. J., Henry, W. L. and Epstein, S. E. (1975) Comparative left ventricular dimensions in trained athletes. *Ann. Intern. Med.* **82**, 521.

Nettles, J. L. and Linscheid, R. L. (1968) Sterno-clavicular dislocations. *J. Trauma* **8(2)**, 158.

Park, W. M., McCall, I. W., McSweeney, T. and Jones, B. F. (1980) Cervicodorsal injury presenting as sternal fracture. *Clin. Radiol.* **31**, 49.

Paskoff, W. J., Coldman, S. and Cohn, K. (1976) The "athletic heart": prevalence and physiological significance of left ventricular enlargement in distance runners. *J. Am. Med. Ass.* **236**, 158.

Petras, A. and Hofman, E. P. (1983) Roentgeno-graphic skeletal injury patterns in parachute jumping. *Am. J. Sports Med.* **11**, 325.

Rasad, S. (1974) Golfer's fractures of the ribs. *Am J. Radiol.* **120**, 901.

Savastano, A. A. and Stutz, S. J. (1978) Traumatic sternoclavicular dislocation. *Int. Surg.* **63**, 10.

Scharplatz, D., Thurleman, K. and Enderlin, F. (1978) Thoracoabdominal trauma in ski accidents. *Injury* **10**, 86.

Scheuer, J. and Tipton, C. M. (1977) Cardiovascular adaptations to physical training. *Ann. Rev. Physiol.* **39**, 221.

Sergent, T. (1973) Major sports injuries. *Practitioner* **210**, 217.

Wakamoto, K. (1969) Electrocardiograms of 25 marathon runners before and after 100 meter dash. *Jpn. Circ. J.* **33**, 105.

4 The Lumbar Spine

Back problems are common in sports such as gymnastics, rowing and weight-lifting as well as in the so-called 'brute' sports such as gridiron football, rugby and wrestling. Serious back injuries also occur in more high-risk activities such as hang-gliding, parachuting and motorized cross-country events on snowmobiles, motor cycles and other types of all-terrain vehicle. Acute soft tissue injuries in the thoracolumbar region are common and in the majority of these radiological investigation is undertaken only to rule out underlying bony damage such as stress fractures of the pars interarticularis.

Where fractures of the lumbar spine occur acutely in a sporting activity they are normally due to direct trauma, for instance the fracture of a spinous process. Occasionally transverse processes may be fractured and this injury can be associated with serious damage to soft tissues, particularly the kidneys. Fractures of the vertebral bodies are, generally speaking, uncommon unless the individual has fallen from a height as in rock-climbing or parachuting. On occasions, forced flexion of the spine results in a fracture in the dorsolumbar region. These injuries are often unstable as there is an associated disruption of the interspinous ligament or fracture of the spinous process. Figures 4.1 and 4.2 show such an injury in a 35-year-old rugby player who sustained this fracture in his last match before retirement. All apparent 'crush' fractures of the dorsolumbar junction should be viewed with great suspicion in view of the possibility of instability and the consequent danger to the conus. This injury was unstable and acute dislocation could have occurred if the patient had been moved carelessly. Because of this, internal fixation was undertaken. A common sequel of such injuries is the progressive deformity (an angular kyphosis) illustrated in Figure 4.3, a view of the dorsolumbar spine of a 30-year-old parachutist taken three years after the incident in which the damage occurred.

Most problems that we see affecting the lumbar region in athletes are due to soft tissue injuries, to abnormalities involving the intervertebral disc, or to stress fractures. The pattern of abnormality depends to some extent on the age of the individual. The adolescent presenting with back pain who has been very active athletically is quite likely to have osteochondritis of the vertebral body (Scheuermann's disease). As in most cases of osteochondritis the aetiology is not clear but there does appear to be an increased incidence in young athletes; the case illustrated in Figure 4.4 is of a 15-year-old international class squash player. The vertebral bodies in these young patients are still growing and the ring epiphyses seen on the anterior, superior and inferior borders of the vertebral bodies become damaged, possibly by the contents of the intervertebral disc rupturing. The changes may be quite extensive and are often associated with narrowing of the disc space anteriorly and wedging of the body of the vertebra. Scheuermann's disease commonly heals without any residual deformity, but on occasions it may result in a kyphosis which can persist into adult life as shown in Figures 4.5 and 4.6 of the spine of a 25-year-old boxer. Similar changes can be seen in interosseous disc herniations, although the localized nature of the deformity should enable infection to be excluded; the appearances are not really consistent with neoplasia.

Spondylolysis may be congenital, or acquired as a type of stress fracture of the pars interarticularis. It may be unilateral or bilateral, and can be associated with spina bifida occulta. The commonest site is at the lumbo-sacral junction and if the defect is large it will be visible on a simple lateral coned view (Figure 4.7). This illustration shows a defect

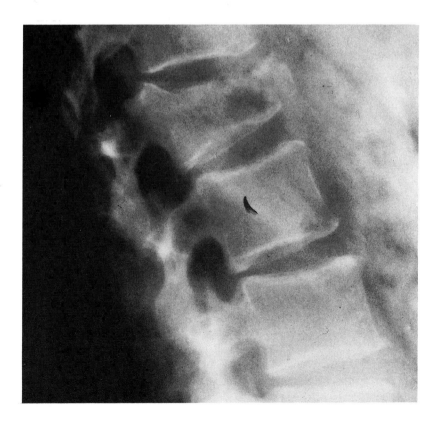

Figure 4.1. Lateral localized view of the lumbar vertebrae showing a fracture of the body of L1.

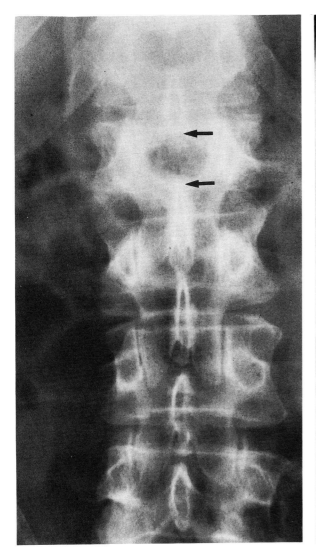

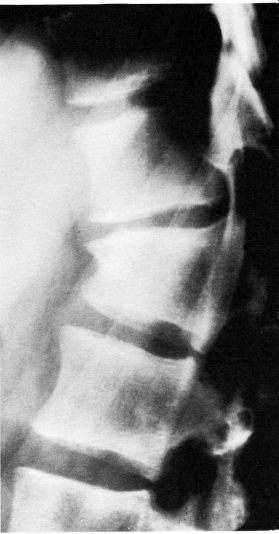

at the L5 level and was found in a 22-year-old rugby player who noted the onset of back pain while playing on hard grounds in South Africa. Figure 4.8 is an oblique of the lumbar spine, and this is the best view to demonstrate the defect, which again is at the L5 level and was found in a 25-year-old West Indian fast bowler who had a very 'whippy' action that put a great deal of stress on this region.

If the initial X-rays are thought to be normal but symptoms persist then an isotope bone scan is a useful screening test to pick out occult lesions. If a recent spondylolysis is present, there will be abnormal activity in the region as is seen in Figure 4.9. This scan was performed in a 14-year-old female high jumper who was complaining of predominantly right-sided lower back pain which settled with rest and rehabilitative physiotherapy but which later recurred, although on the second occasion it involved the left side. Review of these films, together

Figure 4.2. (Above left). Anteroposterior view of the same area as illustrated in Figure 4.1. The widening of the interspinous gap between the spinous processes of D12 and L1 indicates that this is an unstable fracture.

Figure 4.3. (Above right). Lateral view of the dorsolumbar junction showing an angular kyphosis due to an old fracture of the vertebral body of L1 with disruption of the posterior elements which has led to progressive deformity.

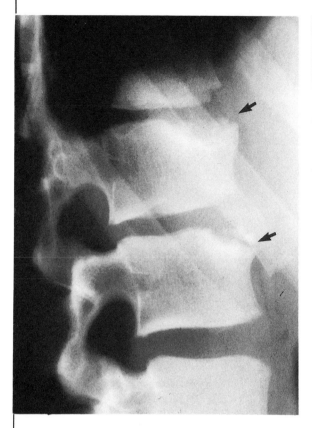

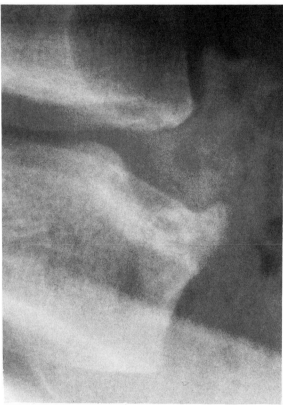

Figure 4.4. (Above left). Lateral view of the lumbar spine in an adolescent showing gross irregularity of the anterior superior borders of two vertebral bodies due to Scheuermann's disease.

Figure 4.5. (Above right). Coned lateral view of a lumbar vertebra showing an extensive anterior deformity of the vertebral body due to old Scheuermann's disease. These appearances would also be compatible with an intra-osseous disc herniation.

with the initial X-rays or further views, may then show an abnormality. However, it must be emphasized that isotope bone scanning is a non-specific test even though it has a high sensitivity for abnormalities. Occasionally spondylolysis gives rise to a secondary sclerosis as illustrated in Figure 4.10 which shows an anteroposterior view of the lower lumbar spine of a 24-year-old fast bowler who complained of persistent back pain throughout the season. Oblique views showed a defect in the pars at this level.

Such stress fractures appear to be common in fast bowlers who perform at a high level, and we have also seen them in many other sports. Figure 4.11 is one of a series of tomograms of the spine of a 28-year-old second row forward who was forced to return home from an overseas tour to New Zealand with back pain. With only conservative management he returned to playing international rugby within eight months.

Spondylolysis is commonest at the L5 level but it can occur higher and at multiple levels. Figure 4.12 shows the spine of a young soccer player from Saudi Arabia who has defects at three levels. This condition would not be helped by his playing on surfaces that are permanently sun-baked and hard.

Where a bilateral spondylolysis allows the vertebral body to slip forward, the condition becomes a spondylolisthesis. The slip clearly causes the intervertebral disc to become disrupted and over a period of years the disc space is lost (Figure 4.13). Eventually, because of this abnormality, the disc above the spondylolisthesis may also be damaged. The case illustrated in Figure 4.13 occurred in a 36-year-old rugby player.

Progressive slipping is extremely uncommon in the mature skeleton. The main danger period appears to be during active growth as is seen in Figure 4.14 which shows severe slippage in a young gymnast. This may be progressive and may result in serious neurological sequelae unless dealt with by fusion of the spine. Surgical intervention in simple spondylolysis is not usually needed unless symptoms are severe and persistent, in which case a Buck's fusion associated with posterior grafting is the normal practice in Cardiff, as has been undertaken in this 24-year-old gymnast (Figure 4.15).

Damage to intervertebral discs in otherwise normal spines is in our experience uncommon in children and adolescents. It does, however, become a problem in young adults, and the incidence increases with age. Fortunately most of these cases have a normal spinal configuration so that investigation by computerized tomography is a simple procedure. We feel it is not warranted to perform myelography as a primary investigation since CT readily demonstrates herniation of disc material and its accuracy is well documented. Most of the problems are lateral disc herniations involving one nerve root as is shown in Figure 4.16

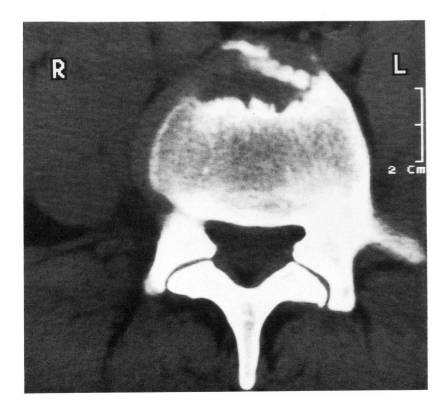

Figure 4.6. CT scan through the superior end-plate of a lumbar vertebra. There is an extensive anterior defect due to Scheuermann's disease.

in this cut through the lumbar spine in a 27-year-old prop forward. Even quite small herniations, such as the one demonstrated in Figure 4.17 in the spine of a 34-year-old weight-lifter, can be readily diagnosed. The ability to investigate these cases in a non-invasive way is a major advance.

The commonest disc damaged in everyday life is at the L5/S1 level, then to a lesser extent at L4/5 and only rarely higher up the spine. There is no doubt, however, that excessive sporting activity can lead to extensive cumulative damage to discs throughout the region, with the inevitable long-term sequelae associated with such deterioration. Figure 4.18 shows the spine of a 45-year-old ex-county class fast bowler now working as a physical education teacher who was having considerable problems related to his back, consequent upon damage he had sustained in a 15-year-long sporting career.

As MRI becomes more widely available, accurate diagnosis in patients with back problems such as disc herniations becomes simpler, as we see in Figure 4.19 which is a lateral view of the spine of a young athlete. One major advantage of this technique is that damage to a disc can be recognized before herniation has occurred, so that the patient need not be subjected to repeated radiological investigation.

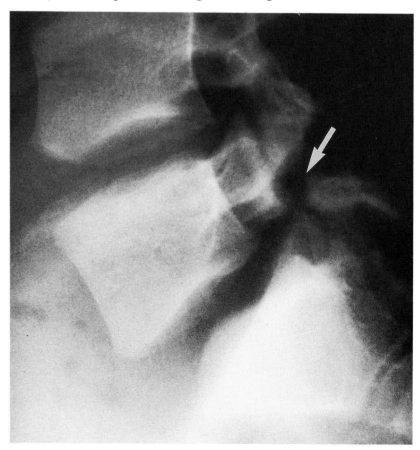

Figure 4.7. Lateral coned view of the lumbosacral junction showing an obvious defect of the pars interarticularis of L5 (spondylolysis).

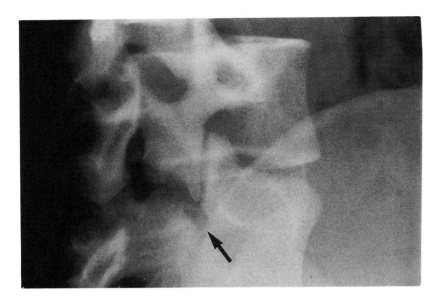

Figure 4.8. Oblique coned view of the lumbosacral junction demonstrating a defect in the pars interarticularis.

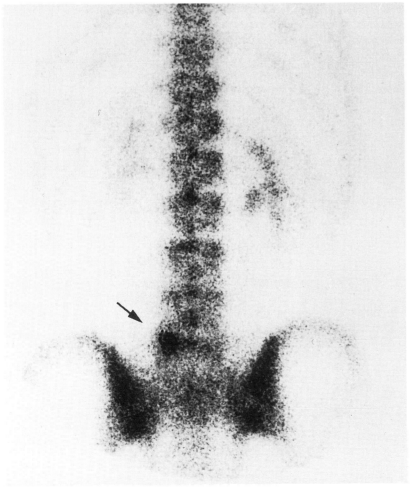

Figure 4.9. Bone scan of the spine and pelvis showing normal activity in the spine and sacroiliac regions but with an abnormally hot area on the right side of L5 indicating localized pathology.

39

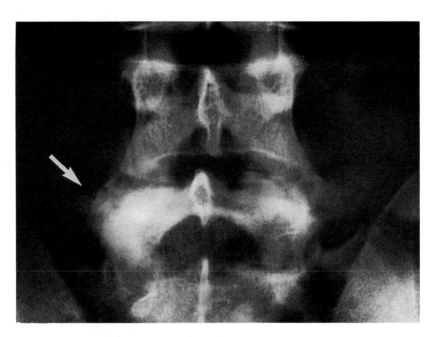

Figure 4.10. (Right). Anteroposterior view of the fifth lumbar vertebra showing abnormal sclerosis on the right side.

Figure 4.11. (Below left). Tomography of the L5 vertebra in the oblique position demonstrating a spondylolysis.

Figure 4.12. (Below right). Oblique view of the lumbar spine showing pars interarticularis defects at three levels.

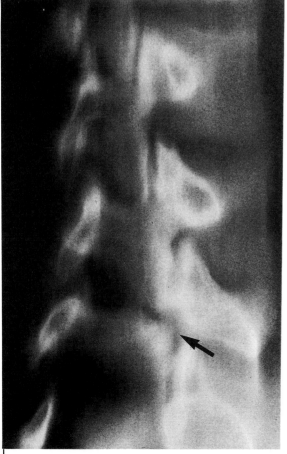

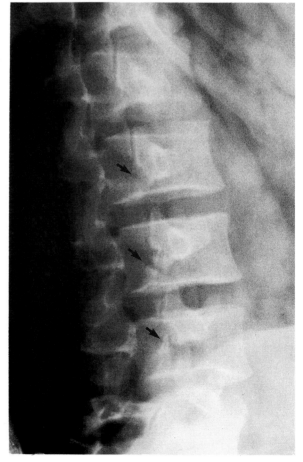

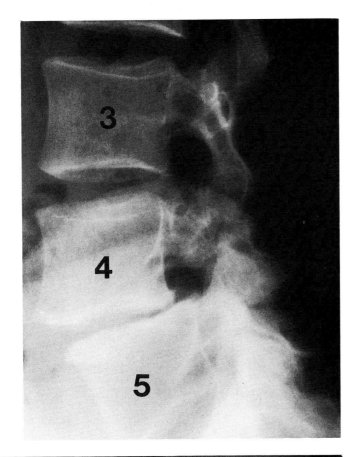

Figure 4.13. Coned view of the L4/5 region showing a degenerative disc with a grade 1 spondylolisthesis.

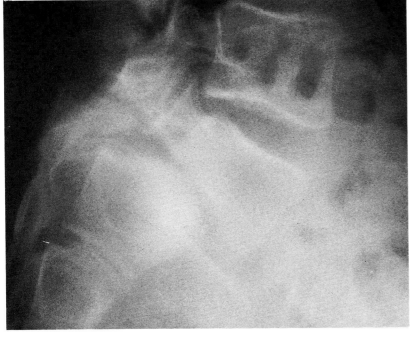

Figure 4.14. Lateral view of the lumbosacral spine in an adolescent showing a severe spondylolisthesis.

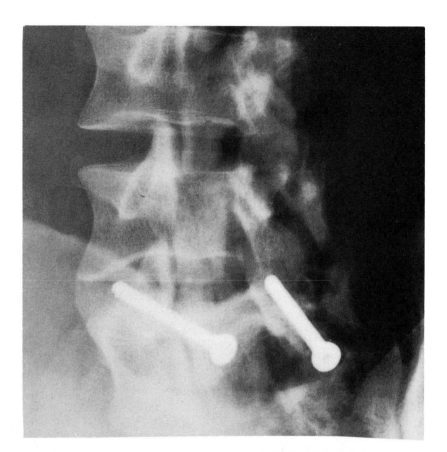

Figure 4.15. Bilateral screw fixation of a spondylolysis.

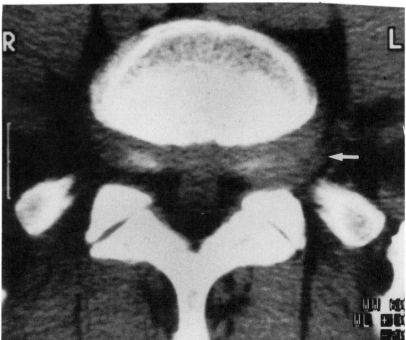

Figure 4.16. CT scan showing a large lateral disc herniation compressing the nerve root on the left.

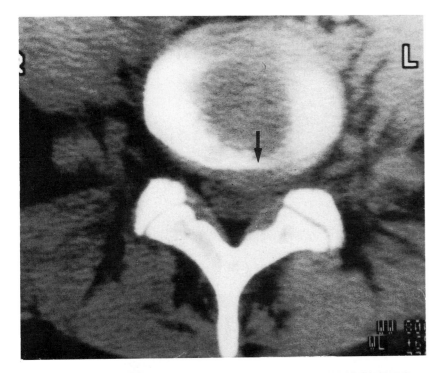

Figure 4.17. CT scan showing a small central–lateral disc herniation with some compression of the theca and left nerve root.

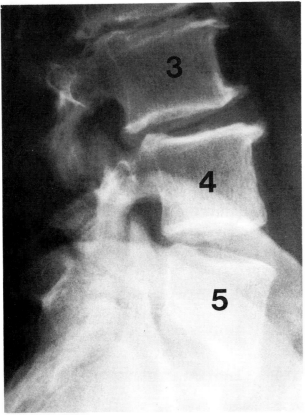

Figure 4.18. Lateral lumbar spine showing gross spondylotic changes with degenerative discs and osteophytes at L2/3 and L3/4.

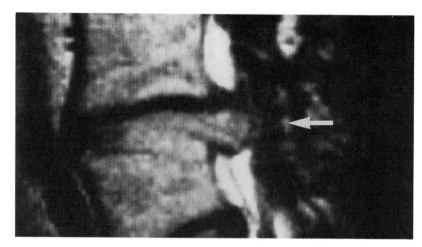

Figure 4.19. Lateral MRI scan demonstrating a large central disc herniation.

● BIBLIOGRAPHY ●

Abel, M. S. (1984) The radiology of low back pain associated with posterior element lesions of the lumbar spine. *CRC Crit. Rev. Diag. Imag.* **20**, 311.

Chafetz, N. I., Mani, J. R., Genant, H. K., *et al.* (1985) CT in low back pain syndrome. *Orthop. Clin. N. Am.* **16**, 395.

Chism, S. E. and Soule, A. B. (1969) Snowmobile injuries: hazards from a popular new winter sport. *J. Am. Med. Ass.* **209**, 1672.

Cyron, B. M., Hutton, W. C. and Troup, J. D. G. (1976) Spondylolytic fractures. *J. Bone Joint Surg.* **58(B)**, 462.

Cyron, B. M. and Hutton, W. C. (1978) The fatigue strength of the lumbar neural arch in spondylolysis. *J. Bone Joint Surg.* **60(B)**, 234.

Davis, M. W., Litman, T., Drill, F. E. and Mueller, J. K. (1977) Ski injuries. *J. Trauma* **17**, 802.

Deutsch, S. D. and Gandsman, E. J. (1983) The use of bone scanning for the diagnosis and management of musculoskeletal trauma. *Surg. Clin. N. Am.* **63(3)**, 567.

Dowling, P. A. (1982) Prospective study of injuries in United States Ski Association freestyle skiing—1976-77 and 1979-80. *Am. J. Sports Med.* **10**, 268.

Dubowitz, B., Friedman, L. and Papert, B. (1987) The oblique cranial tilt view for spondylolysis. *J. Bone Joint Surg.* **69(B)**, 421.

Elliott, S., Hutson, M. A. and Wastie, M. L. (1988) Bone scintigraphy in the assessment of spondylolysis in patients attending a Sports Injury Clinic. *Clin. Radiol.* **39(3)**, 269.

Fahrni, W. H. and Trueman, G. E. (1965) Comparative radiological study of spines of a primitive population with North Americans and Northern Europeans. *J. Bone Joint Surg.* **47(B)**, 552.

Farfan, H. F., Osteria, V. and Lamy, C. (1976) The mechanical etiology of spondylolysis and spondylolisthesis. *Clin. Orthop.* **117**, 40.

Ferguson, R. J. (1974) Low back pain in college football linemen. *J. Bone Joint Surg.* **56(A)**, 1300.

Keene, J. S. (1987) Thoraco-lumbar fractures in winter sports. *Clin. Orthop.* **216**, 39.

Lysholm, J. and Wiklander, J. (1987) Injuries in runners. *Am. J. Sports Med.* **15**, 168.

Margreiter, R., Raas, E. and Lugger, L. J. (1976) The risk of injury in experienced alpine skiers. *Orthop. Clin. N. Am.* **7**, 51.

Micheli, L. J. (1979) Low back pain in the adolescent: differential diagnosis. *Am. J. Sports Med.* **7**, 362.

Micheli, L. J. (1983) Back injuries in dancers. *Clin. Sports Med.* **2**, 473.

Modic, M. T. and Weinstein, M. A. (1984) Nuclear magnetic resonance of the spine. *Br. Med. Bull.* **40**, 183.

Modic, M. T., Masaryk, T., Boumphrey, F., Goormastic, M., and Bell, G. (1986) Lumbar herniated disk disease and canal stenosis: Prospective evaluation of surface coil M.R., C.T., and Myelography. *Am. J. Radiol.* **147**, 757.

Newman, P. H. (1963) The etiology of spondylolisthesis. *J. Bone Joint Surg.* **45(B)**, 39.

Papanicolaou, N., Wilkinson, R. H., Emans, J. B., Treves, S. and Micheli, L. J. (1985) Bone scintigraphy and radiology in young athletes with low back pain. *Am. J. Radiol.* **145**, 1039.

Pedersen, A. K. and Hagen, R. (1988) Spondylolysis and spondylolisthesis. *J. Bone Joint Surg.* **70(A)**, 15.

Porter, R. W. and Park, W. (1982) Unilateral spondylolysis. *J. Bone Joint Surg.* **64(B)**, 344.

Porter, R. W. and Hibbert, C. S. (1984) Symptoms associated with lysis of the pars interarticularis. *Spine* **9(7)**, 755.

Ramirez, L. F. and Javid, M. J. (1985) Cost effectiveness of chemonucleolysis versus laminectomy in treatment of herniated nucleus pulposus. *Spine* **10**, 363.

Rombold, C. (1966) Treatment of spondylolisthesis by posterolateral fusion, resection of the pars interarticularis, and prompt mobilization of the patient. *J. Bone Joint Surg.* **48(B)**, 1282.

Schipper, J., Kardaun, J. W. P. F., Braakman, R., *et al.* (1987) Lumbar disk herniation: diagnosis with CT or Myelography. *Radiology* **165**, 227.

Schneiderman, G., *et al.* (1987) Magnetic resonance imaging in the diagnosis of disc degeneration: correlation with discography. *Spine* **12**, 276.

Spincer, C. W. III and Jackson, D. W. (1983) Back injuries in the athlete. *Clin. Sports Med.* **2**, 191.

Steinberg, P. J. (1988) Injuries to Dutch sports parachutists. *B. J. Sports Med.* **22**, 25.

Stoddard, A. and Osborn, J. F. (1979) Scheuermann's disease or spinal osteochondrosis. *J. Bone Joint Surg.* **61(B)**, 56.

Fredrickson, B. E., Baker, D., McHolick, W. J., Yuan, H. A. and Lubicky, J. P. (1984) The natural history of spondylolysis and spondylolisthesis. *J. Bone Joint Surg.* **66(A)**, 699.

Frymoyer, J. W. and Pope, M. H. (1978) The role of trauma in low back pain: a review. *J. Trauma* **18**, 628.

Frymoyer, J. W., Pope, M. H. and Costanza, M. C., *et al.* (1980) Epidemiologic studies of low-back pain. *Spine* **5**, 419.

Gibson, M. J., Buckley, J., Mawhinney, R., Mulholland, R. C. and Worthington, B. S. (1986) Magnetic resonance imaging and discography in the diagnosis of disc degeneration. *J. Bone Joint Surg.* **68(B)**, 369.

Gibson, M. J., Szypryt, E. P., Buckley, J. H., Worthington, B. S. and Mulholland, R. C. (1987) Magnetic resonance imaging of adolescent disc herniation. *J. Bone Joint Surg.* **69(B)**, 699.

Greenhough, C. G., Dimmock, S., Edwards, D., Ransford, A., and Bentley, G. (1986) The role of computerised tomography in intervertebral disc prolapse. *J. Bone Joint Surg.* **68(B)**, 729.

Grogan, J. P., *et al.* (1982) Spondylolysis studied at computed tomography. *Radiology* **145**, 737.

Gutman, J., Weisbuch, J. and Wolf, M. (1974) Ski injuries in 1972-73: report analysis of a major health program. *J. Am. Med. Ass.* **230**, 1423.

Hadler, N. M. (1987) Regional musculoskeletal disease of the low back: cumulative trauma versus single incident. *Clin. Orthop.* **221**, 33.

Haughton, V. M. (1988) M.R. Imaging of the spine. *Radiology* **166**, 297.

Hill, G. M. and Ellis, E. A. (1987) Chemonucleolysis as an alternative to laminectomy for the herniated lumbar disc. *Clin. Orthop.* **225**, 229.

Holdsworth, F. (1970) Fractures, dislocations and fracture–dislocations of the spine. *J. Bone Joint Surg.* **52(A)**, 1534.

Hoshina, H. (1980) Spondylolysis in athletes. *Phys. Sportsmed.* **8**, 75.

Ireland, M. and Micheli, L. J. (1987) Bilateral stress fracture of the lumbar pedicles in a ballet dancer: a case report. *J. Bone Joint Surg.* **69(A)**, 140.

Jackson, D. W., Wiltse, L. L. and Cirincione, R. J. (1976) Spondylolysis in the female gymnast. *Clin. Orthop.* **117**, 68.

Keene, J. S. (1983) Low back pain in athletes from spondylogenic injury during recreation or competition. *Postgrad. Med.* **74**, 209.

Keene, J. S. (1984) Radiographic evaluation of thoracolumbar fractures. *Clin. Orthop.* **189**, 58.

Van den Oever, M., Merrick, M. V. and Scott, J. H. S. (1987) Bone scintigraphy in symptomatic spondylolysis. *J. Bone Joint Surg.* **69(B)**, 453.

Williams, A. L., Haughton, W. M., Meyer, G. A. and Ho, K. C. (1982) The computed tomographic appearance of the bulging annulus. *Radiology* **142**, 403.

Withingon, R. L. and Hall, L. W. (1970). Snowmobile accidents: a review of injuries sustained in the use of snowmobiles in northern New England during the 1968-69 season. *J. Trauma* **10**, 760.

Wynne-Davies, R. and Scott, J. H. W. (1979) Inheritance and spondylolisthesis: a radiographic family survey. *J. Bone Joint Surg.* **61(B)**, 301.

5 The Shoulder

Shoulder problems are particularly common in sports such as swimming, tennis and rowing, as well as in the contact sports where heavy falls occur frequently. On average, injuries to this area make up about ten per cent of a sports medicine practice.

The bone in the shoulder girdle that fractures most often is the clavicle, as shown in Figure 5.1 which illustrates a displaced fracture in a 28-year-old rugby player who was heavily tackled onto his right side. Such fractures are easily diagnosed clinically as they can be both seen and felt, and X-rays are taken only to document the injury and to assess the degree of displacement. In some centres, if there is marked displacement, treatment is by internal fixation but the vast majority of clavicular fractures are managed conservatively.

Injuries to the acromioclavicular joint can also be assessed clinically, particularly where the joint is dislocated. However, subluxation can be more difficult to diagnose as, when acute, the deformity may be masked by soft tissue swelling. Films taken with the patient holding a heavy weight on the injured side usually demonstrate the lesion quite clearly when the arm is pulled down, as is seen in Figure 5.2 which shows the left shoulder of a 23-year-old soccer player. Occasionally these injuries are fracture–dislocations, the fracture involving the outer aspect of the clavicle, and this results in a residual deformity and often persistent discomfort.

Figure 5.3 is a radiograph of the distal portion of the right clavicle of a 34-year-old rugby league player. It shows the appearances produced by an old injury to the acromioclavicular joint that was severe enough to damage the coracoclavicular ligament, which has subsequently ossified.

Figure 5.4 is a view of the left clavicle of a 31-year-old man who injured his shoulder two years previously in a judo competition. Again, extensive ossification is seen in the coracoclavicular ligament which was badly damaged at the time. Where there has been recurrent damage to the joint, as illustrated in the radiograph of the left shoulder of a 41-year-old rugby player, degenerative changes occur as illustrated in Figure 5.5. This man presented with episodic pain and stiffness in the joint

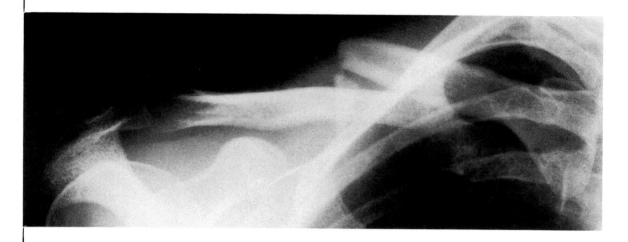

Figure 5.1. Displaced fracture of the right clavicle.

which interfered with his heavy manual work in the coal mining industry. An occasional sequel to significant or recurrent damage to the distal clavicle is osteolysis, which also sometimes occurs in weight-lifters (Figure 5.6) and other athletes who engage in a lot of upper body work.

Osteochondral fractures of the glenohumeral joint may result in the release of bone marrow containing fat into the joint. If the subsequent X-rays are taken with the patient in the erect position, a fluid level may be seen (Figure 5.7). Aspiration of the joint under these circumstances demonstrates the presence of a lipohaemarthrosis. This unpleasant fracture to the humeral neck was sustained by a 42-year-old man who came off his horse while fox-hunting. When a lipohaemarthrosis has been noted and no fracture is immediately obvious, further views should be taken and examined carefully; if necessary the joint should be screened for an osteochondral fracture. These fractures may be quite small (Figure 5.8) but they do indicate severe damage to the joint. The case illustrated is that of a 28-year-old physiotherapist who injured her left shoulder while skiing. The fragment involved resulted in an impingement syndrome with pain and limitation of shoulder movement, and surgical intervention was subsequently needed. Larger osteochondral fragments may become completely detached within the joint as is illustrated in Figure 5.9 in the right shoulder of a 34-year-old rugby player. This fragment was removed surgically. Where clinical suspicion of an osteochondral fracture is high, and if such a lesion has not been demonstrated by conventional X-rays or by screening, CT scanning can be helpful (Figure 5.9).

Fractures lower down the humeral shaft are occasionally seen in the 'brute' sports and sometimes also as stress-related phenomena, such as the one illustrated in Figure 5.10 which occurred spontaneously in a 15-year-old baseball pitcher while he was throwing. There was no evidence of any pathological bone disorder.

The glenohumeral joint may dislocate anteriorly, posteriorly or occasionally inferiorly. Most commonly the displaced humerus comes

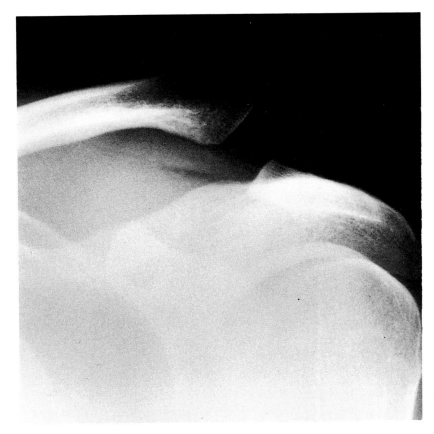

Figure 5.2. (Left). Acute acromio-clavicular dislocation.

Figure 5.3. (Below). Old injury to the acromioclavicular joint. The deformity of the end of the clavicle indicates an associated fracture and there is also some ossification of the coracoclavicular ligament (arrow).

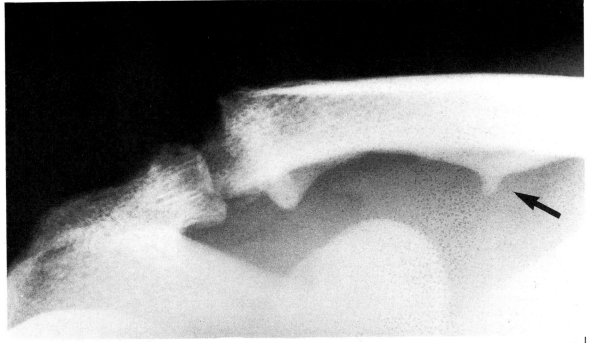

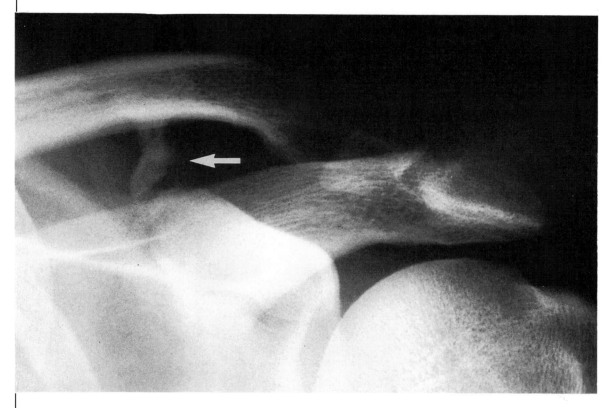

Figure 5.4. Extensive ossification of the coracoclavicular ligament due to previous injury.

to lie anterior to the glenoid beneath the coracoid process. The diagnosis can usually be made on clinical grounds, given the abnormal appearances of the injured shoulder, although this may be more difficult in heavily muscled individuals. The anteroposterior view of the shoulder is diagnostic (Figure 5.11) and it is not necessary to subject the patient to further uncomfortable X-ray examinations to produce axial views, although a trans-scapular view may be useful. When the anteroposterior film is thought to be normal or equivocal, the presence of a posterior dislocation should be considered. Many posterior dislocations result from an abnormal muscular contraction, for instance as the result of an electric shock, but they are seen secondary to trauma. The anterior view of the shoulder may be quite normal, although an axial view (Figure 5.12) will demonstrate the head of the humerus lying posterior to the glenoid. Due to muscular spasm and pain it may sometimes be necessary to give the patient sedation and/or analgesia in order to obtain adequate films.

Disruption of the rotator cuff and capsule may lead to inferior subluxation of the shoulder (Figure 5.13) as seen in this 28-year-old gymnast who presented with a past history of several injuries to his left shoulder. This injury may not be apparent on routine films but can readily be demonstrated on screening the sedated patient.

A diagnostic problem that is commonly met in athletes, particularly gymnasts, is the 'clicking' or 'clunking' shoulder, the patient stating that their 'shoulder comes out'. When the diagnosis of true dislocation can be confirmed, good results may be expected from surgical repair, but this is not so if the patient has had many previous episodes of dislocation, as a false joint with severe deformity of the glenoid and the head of the humerus can sometimes develop (Figure 5.14) as has happened in this 35-year-old wrestler. Clearly this is an unsatisfactory situation and the diagnosis should have been made far earlier since the plain film findings are usually quite obvious provided that appropriate views are obtained. As the commonest problem is one of recurrent anterior dislocation, the lesion appears on the posterior surface of the head of the humerus and on the anterior surface of the glenoid. The defect that develops on the humeral head (Hill–Sachs or hatchet defect) is best demonstrated by taking a radiograph with the arm internally rotated so that the posterior surface of the head of the humerus comes on to the skyline, as is shown in Figure 5.15 in the right shoulder of a 32-year-old rugby player. Another sensitive method of assessing this lesion is to screen the affected shoulder using image intensification. Smaller lesions can be identified using this technique, as is seen in Figure 5.16 which demonstrates the problem in a 26-year-old soccer player who was able to continue active participation after surgery.

The inferior cartilaginous rim of the glenoid is also damaged in patients with recurrent anterior dislocation. This produces the so-called Bankart's lesion which is not normally visible on routine views. However, when the damage is more extensive, the underlying bone becomes irregular and new bone formation may occur (Figure 5.17) as is seen in this lesion in the right shoulder of a 25-year-old cricketer. These defects can also be demonstrated by arthrography, CT, or a combination of both techniques and Figure 5.18, a CT of the normal shoulder is included for comparison purposes. CT of the shoulder without contrast medium can, in itself, be useful and the anatomical cross-section demonstrated enables small bony lesions to be readily diagnosed, as in this view of the shoulder of a 30-year-old cricketer (Figure 5.19) who subsequently

Figure 5.5. Irregularity of the acromioclavicular joint due to previous trauma with multiple small bony fragments in the soft tissues.

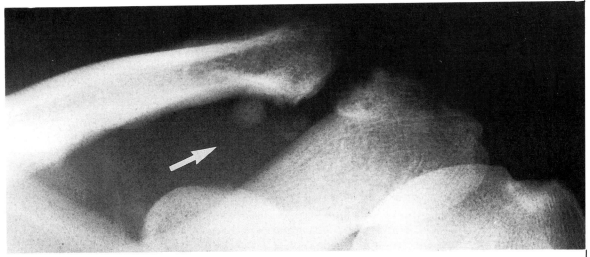

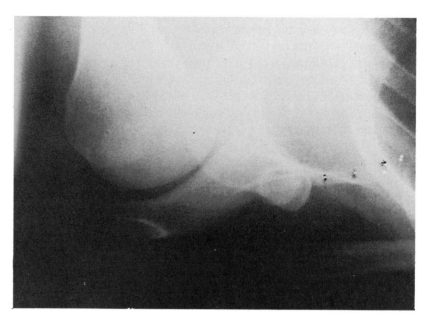

Figure 5.6. Radiograph of the left shoulder demonstrating osteolysis of the distal clavicle produced by weight-lifting.

underwent surgical repair of his damaged and recurrently dislocating joint. Larger osteochondral defects are even easier to demonstrate as shown in the scan (Figure 5.20) of the left shoulder of a 31-year-old rugby player who had dislocated his shoulder four times in a month, following an initial injury sustained while playing on hard pitches in Florida.

Arthography of the shoulder, whether single or double contrast techniques are used, can be valuable, as the glenoid labrum and articular cartilage can be shown. Figure 5.21 is a double contrast arthrogram of the left shoulder of a 25-year-old tennis player; the presence of a full thickness tear of the capsule is recognized by the contrast medium entering the subacromial bursa. More recently it has been suggested that a combination of arthrography and CT will supply even more information, although our experience of this technique is limited.

Osteoarthritis of the shoulder joint may develop in individuals who have had recurrent trauma to the joint and is readily recognized since its appearances are similar to that of the condition in other joints, *e.g.* loss of articular cartilage, sclerosis of the bone ends, subarticular cysts and osteophyte formation. Figure 5.22 is the right shoulder of a 38-year-old former fast bowler, and illustrates the type of problem that can occur, although fortunately the development of this painful condition is not as common as in the weight-bearing joints of the lower limb.

Another degenerative phenomenon related to the severe wear and tear to which some athletes subject their shoulders is calcification in the supraspinatus tendon (Figure 5.23) which is illustrated in this view of the shoulder of a 31-year-old oarswoman who presented with an acutely stiff and painful shoulder the day after a nine-mile row. The condition responded satisfactorily to local corticosteroid injection.

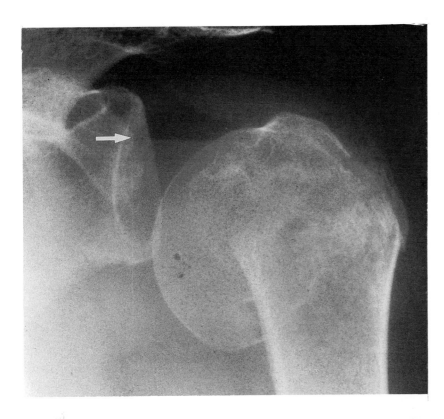

Figure 5.7. (Left). Fracture of the neck of the humerus with inferior subluxation of the head of the humerus and a fluid level (arrow) within the joint. This fluid level represents a lipohaemarthrosis (see text).

Figure 5.8. (Below). Small osteochondral fracture (arrow).

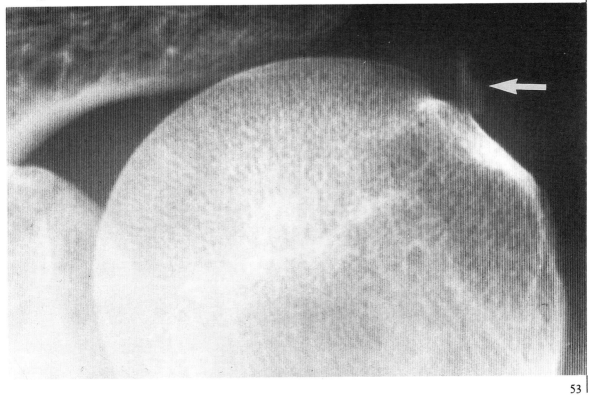

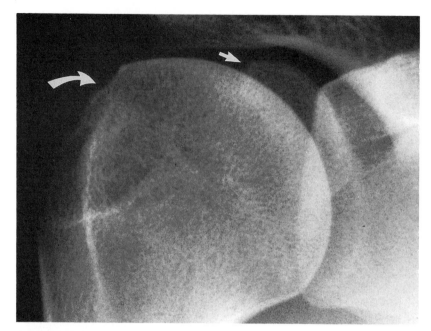

Figure 5.9. Osteochondral fracture of the head of the humerus with a large intra-articular loose body (small arrow). The fracture site is marked by a curved arrow.

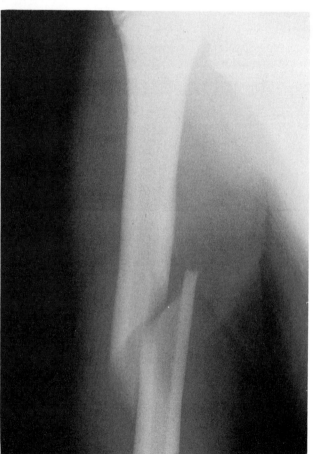

Figure 5.10. Spontaneous displaced spiral fracture of the mid-shaft of the humerus in a 15-year-old boy.

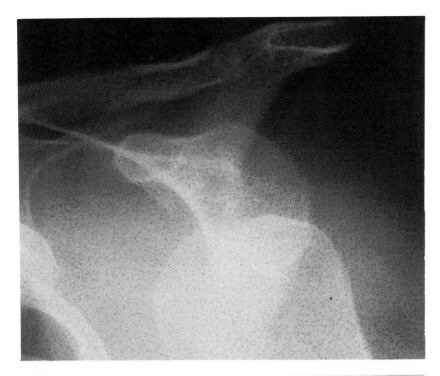

Figure 5.11. Anteroposterior view of the shoulder showing an anterior dislocation in a 22-year-old soccer player. An axial view is not necessary.

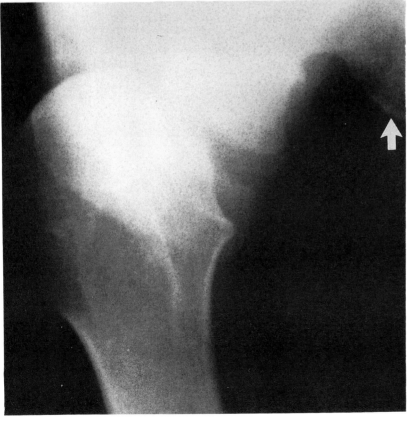

Figure 5.12. Axial view of the shoulder showing a posterior dislocation. The coracoid process lying anterior to the glenoid is arrowed.

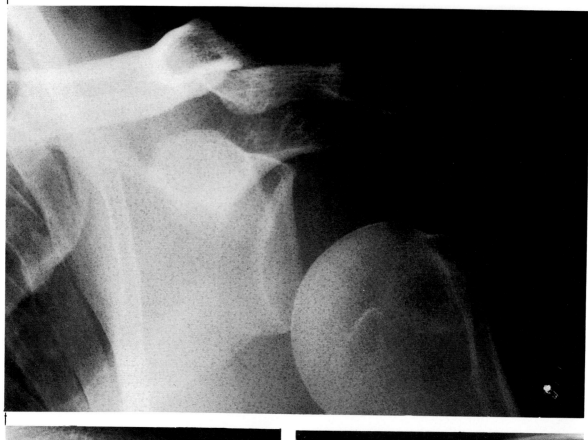

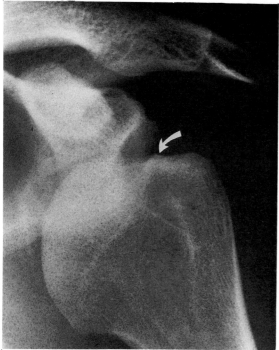
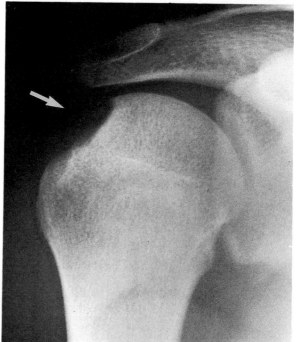

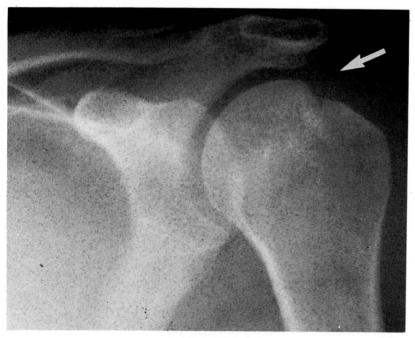

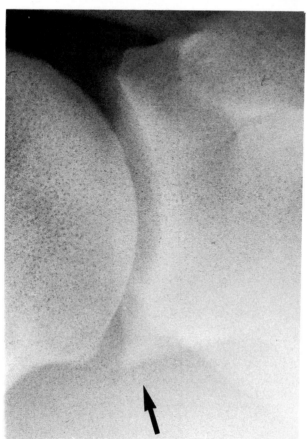

Figure 5.13. (Facing top). Inferior subluxation of the head of the humerus. There is an associated fracture of the clavicle.

Figure 5.14. (Facing bottom left). Anterior dislocation of the shoulder. This is a recurrent problem in this patient. Note the deformities of the glenoid and the head of the humerus (arrow).

Figure 5.15. (Facing bottom right). There is a large defect in the head of the humerus, the so-called Hill–Sachs lesion which is arrowed. This is due to recurrent anterior dislocation with impingement of the head of the humerus on the anterior surface of the glenoid.

Figure 5.16. (Above left). A small but obvious Hill–Sachs lesion (arrow) due to recurrent anterior dislocation.

Figure 5.17. (Left). Enlarged oblique view of the glenoid, showing new bone formation at the inferior border of the glenoid (arrow) due to recurrent dislocation.

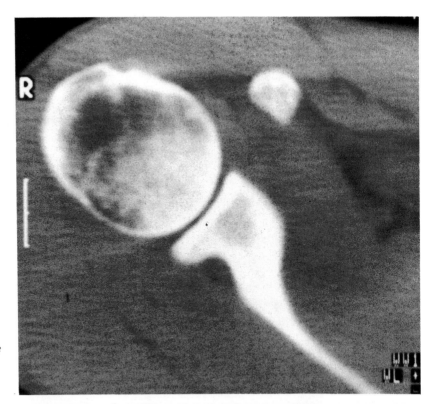

Figure 5.18. CT scan of a
normal shoulder. Note the
round head of humerus and the
normal glenoid. The fragment
of bone seen anteriorly is the
tip of the coracoid process.

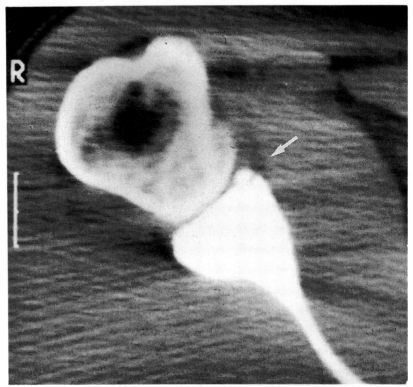

Figure 5.19. CT scan of a
shoulder showing a small
osteochondral fracture (arrow)
of the glenoid due to recurrent
anterior dislocation.

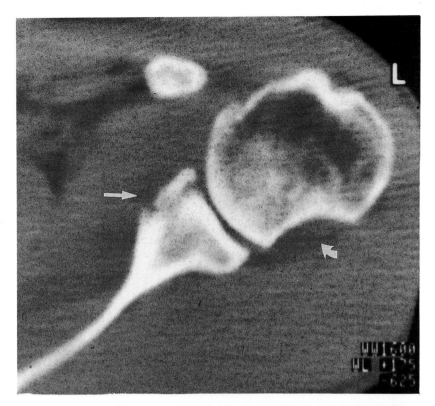

Figure 5.20. CT scan of a shoulder showing a large osteochondral defect of the anterior border of the glenoid (straight arrow). The bone fragment lying in the soft tissues is a normal coracoid process. There is a large defect in the head of the humerus (curved arrow). This is a Hill-Sachs lesion.

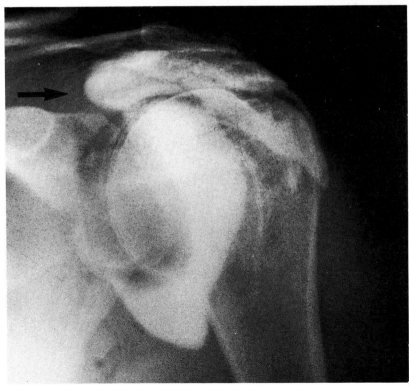

Figure 5.21. Double contrast shoulder arthrogram. There is filling of the subacromial bursa (arrow) indicating a full thickness tear of the capsule of the joint.

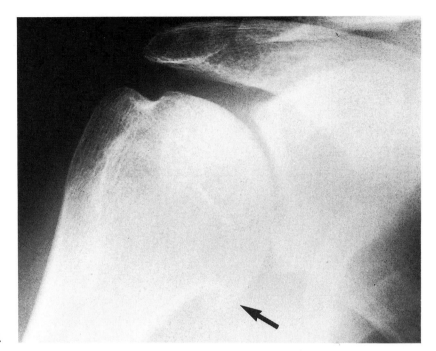

Figure 5.22. Osteoarthritis of the shoulder joint due to recurrent trauma. Note the narrowing of the joint due to loss of articular cartilage and the osteophyte on the inferior border of the humerus (arrow).

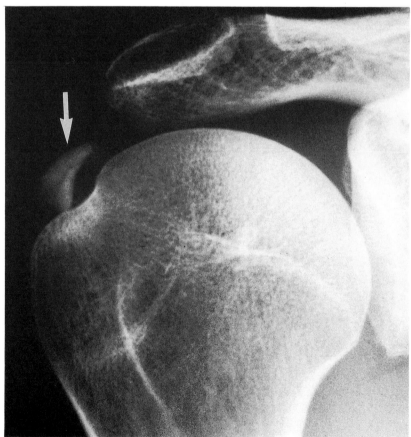

Figure 5.23. Calcification of supraspinatus tendon in a 31-year-old oarswoman.

● BIBLIOGRAPHY ●

Andrews, J. R., Carson, W. G. and McLeod, W. D. (1985) Glenoid labrum tears related to the long head of the biceps. *Am. J. Sports Med.* **13**, 337.

Arndt, J. H. and Sears, A. D. (1965) Posterior dislocation of the shoulder. *Am. J. Radiol.* **94**, 639.

Bankart, A. S. B. (1923) Recurrent or habitual dislocation of the shoulder joint. *Br. Med. J.* **2**, 1132.

Bankart, A. S. B. (1938) The pathology and treatment of recurrent dislocation of the shoulder joint. *Br. J. Surg.* **26**, 23.

Bateman, J. E. (1962) Athletic injuries about the shoulder in throwing and body contact sports. *Clin. Orthop.* **23**, 75.

Bennett, G. E. (1947) Shoulder and elbow lesions distinctive of baseball players. *Ann. Surg.* **126**, 107.

Blazina, E. and Satzman, J. S. (1969) Recurrent anterior subluxation of the shoulder in athletes: a distinct entity. *J. Bone Joint Surg.* **5(A)**, 1037.

Bost, F. C. and Inman, V. T. (1942) The pathological changes in recurrent dislocation of the shoulder. *J. Bone Joint Surg.* **15**, 595.

Braunstein, E. M. and O'Connor, G. (1982) Double contrast arthrotomography of the shoulder. *J. Bone Joint Surg.* **64(A)**, 192.

Cahill, B. R. (1982) Osteolysis of the distal part of the clavicle in male athletes. *J. Bone Joint Surg.* **64(A)**, 1053.

Carr, D., Johnson, R. J. and Pope, M. H. (1981) Upper extremity injuries in skiing. *Am. J. Sports Med.* **9**, 378.

Cofield, R. H. and Simonet, W. T. (1984) The shoulder in sport. *Mayo Clin. Proc.* **59**, 157.

Cone, R. O. III, Resnick, D. and Danzig, L. (1984) Shoulder impingement syndrome: radiographic evaluation. *Radiology* **150**, 29.

Danzig, L. A., Greenway, G. and Resnick, D. (1980) The Hill–Sachs lesion. *Am. J. Sports Med.* **9**, 328.

Danzig, L. A., Resnick, D. and Greenway, G. (1982) Evaluation of unstable shoulders by CT. *Am. J. Sports Med.* **10**, 138.

Dias, J. J., Steingold, R. F., Richardson, R. A., Tesfayohannes, B. and Gregg, P. J. (1987) The conservative treatment of acromioclavicular dislocations. *J. Bone Joint Surg.* **69(B)**, 719.

Diveley, R. L. and Meyer, P. W. (1959) Baseball shoulder. *J. Am. Med. Ass.* **171**, 1659.

Glick, J. M., Milburn, L. J., Haggerty, J. F. and Nishimoto, D. (1977) Dislocated acromioclavicular joint. Follow-up study of 35 unreduced acromio-clavicular dislocations. *Am. J. Sports Med.* **5**, 264.

Goldman, A. B. and Gleman, B. (1978) The double-contrast shoulder arthogram: a review of 158 studies. *Radiology* **127**, 655.

Hawkins, R. J. and Kennedy, J. C. (1980) Impingement syndrome in athletes. *Am. J. Sports Med.* **8**, 151.

Hill, H. A. and Sachs, M. D. (1940) The grooved defect of the humeral head. *Radiology* **35**, 690.

Jackson, D. W. (1976) Chronic rotation cuff impingement in the throwing athlete. *Am. J. Sports Med.* **4**, 231.

Jobe, F. W. and Jobe, C. M. (1983) Painful athletic injuries of the shoulder. *Clin. Orthop.* **173**, 117.

Kessel, L. (1982) *Clinical Disorders of the Shoulder.* Edinburgh: Churchill Livingstone.

Kleinman, P. K., Kanzaria, P. K., Goss, T. P. and Pappas, A. M. (1984) Axillary arthrotomography of the glenoid labrum. *Am. J. Radiol.* **141**, 993.

Kuriyama, S., Fujimaki. E., Katagiri, T. and Uemura, S. (1984) Anterior dislocation of the shoulder joint sustained through skiing. *Am. J. Sports Med.* **12**, 339.

Levine, A. H., Pias, M. J. and Schwartz, E. E. (1976) Post-traumatic osteolysis of the distal clavicle with emphasis on early radiologic changes. *Am. J. Radiol.* **127**, 781.

McLean, I. D. (1984) Swimmers' injuries. *Aust. Fam. Phys.* **13**, 499.

Morimoto, K., *et al.* (1988) Calcification of the coracoacromial ligament. *Am. J. Sports Med.* **16(1)**, 80.

Moseley, H. F. (1959) Athletic injuries to the shoulder region. *Am. J. Surg.* **98**, 401.

Neer, C. S. II (1972) Anterior acromioplasty for the chronic impingement syndrome of the shoulder. *J. Bone Joint Surg.* **54(A)**, 41.

Neer, C. S. II (1983) Impingement lesion. *Clin. Orthop.* **173**, 70.

Neer, C. S. II and Welsh, R. P. (1977) The shoulder in sports. *Orthop. Clin. N. Am.* **9**, 583.

Neer, C. S. II, Craig, E. V. and Fukuda, H. (1983) Cuff-tear arthropathy. *J. Bone Joint Surg.* **65(A)**, 1232.

Neviaser, T. J. (1980) Arthrography of the shoulder. *Orthop. Clin. N. Am.* **11**, 205.

Neviaser, R. J. and Neviaser, T. J. (1987) The frozen shoulder: diagnosis and management. *Clin. Orthop.* **223**, 59.

Pappas, A. M., Goss, T. P. and Kleinman, P. K. (1983) Symptomatic shoulder instability due to lesions of the glenoid labrum. *Am. J. Sports Med.* **11**, 279.

Park, J. P., Arnold, J. A., Coker, T. P., Harris, W. D. and Becker, D. A. (1980) Treatment of acromioclavicular separations. A retrospective study. *Am. J. Sports Med.* **8**, 251.

Penny, J. N. and Welsh, R. P. (1981) Shoulder impingement syndromes in athletes and their surgical management. *Am. J. Sports Med.* **9**, 11.

Post, M. and Cohen, J. (1987) Impingement syndrome: a review of late stage II and early stage III lesions. *Clin. Orthop.* **207**, 126.

Post, M., Silver, R. and Singh, M. (1983) Rotator cuff tear: diagnosis and treatment. *Clin. Orthop.* **173**, 78.

Rafii, M., Firooznia, H., Bonamo, J. J., Bonamo, J. J., Minkhoff, J. and Golimbu, C. (1987) Athlete shoulder injuries: CT arthrographic findings. *Radiology* **162**, 559.

Reeves, B. (1969) Acute anterior dislocation of the shoulder. *Ann. R. Coll. Surg. Engl.* **44**, 255.

Rowe, C. R. and Zarins, B. (1981) Recurrent transient subluxation of the shoulder. *J. Bone Joint Surg.* **63(A)**, 863.

Samilson, R. L. and Prieto, V. (1983) Dislocation arthropathy of the shoulder. *J. Bone Joint Surg.* **65(A)**, 456.

Scott, J. C. and Orr, M. M. (1973) Injuries to the acromioclavicular joint. *Injury* **5**, 13.

Smith, M. J. and Stewart, M. J. (1979) Acute acromioclavicular separations. A 20-year study. *Am. J. Sports Med.* **7**, 62.

Taft, T. N., Wilson, F. C. and Oglesby, J. W. (1987) Dislocation of the acromioclavicular joint. *J. Bone Joint Surg.* **69(A)**, 1045.

Wallace, W. A. and Hellier, M. (1983) Improving radiographs of the injured shoulder. *Radiography* **49**, 229.

Weaver, J. K. (1987) Skiing-related injuries to the shoulder. *Clin. Orthop.* **216**, 24.

6 The Elbow and Forearm

Sports that involve throwing, pitching, bowling and the use of a racquet tend to cause problems at the elbow joint of the dominant arm. The joint is also frequently damaged in contact sports by falls onto its 'point' and onto the outstretched hand. As an example, Figure 6.1 is a lateral view of the joint in a 34-year-old tennis player who fell onto his elbow and sustained this displaced fracture of the olecranon which subsequently required internal fixation.

The commonest site for fractures around the elbow, however, is at the radial head/neck. These injuries are easily missed on X-ray as frequently the only indication of their presence is the haemarthrosis that they cause. Figure 6.2 illustrates such a fracture in a basketball player who fell onto his outstretched hand.

In contact sports more severe injuries may result, and Figure 6.3 shows a posterior dislocation of the elbow in a 24-year-old full-back who sustained this injury in a diving tackle with his arm at full stretch. He was able to return to competitive sport within about two months of the incident.

We have also seen these dislocations in gymnasts, as well as supracondylar fractures such as the one illustrated in Figure 6.4. These injuries always carry with them the risk of potentially crippling neurovascular damage, although fortunately this did not occur in this case.

A direct blow to the forearm can cause an isolated fracture of one of the bones, as can be seen in Figure 6.5. This was sustained by a 31-year-old goalkeeper who was struck on the arm by the boot of an opposing striker as the 'keeper dived in at his feet to make a save.

Whilst we have seen that isolated fractures do occur, it is important that the whole of the forearm including the joints at either end should be carefully inspected clinically and radiologically or dislocations may easily be missed. A classic example is shown in Figure 6.6 which is the lateral view of the forearm of a young cyclist who has sustained a fracture of the mid-shaft of the ulna associated with a dislocation of the proximal radio-ulnar joint, the so-called Monteggia fracture. Similarly

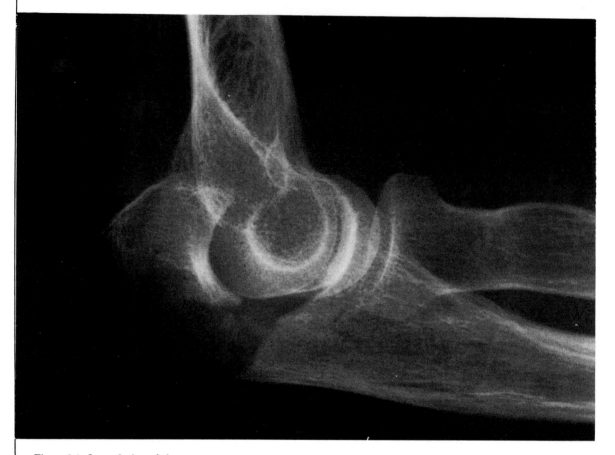

Figure 6.1. Lateral view of the elbow showing a typical displaced fracture of the olecranon.

a fracture of the lower part of the shaft of the radius may be associated with a dislocation of the distal radio-ulnar joint (Galeazzi fracture/dislocation) as is seen in Figure 6.7 which is a film of the forearm of a 25-year-old rugby player.

Where both of the forearm bones are fractured, the wrist and elbow joints are rarely damaged and the degree of displacement makes the fracture very obvious clinically. However, this is not invariable and Figure 6.8 shows comminuted fractures of the radius and ulna together with an associated dislocation of the proximal radio-ulnar joint in a skate-boarder.

Isolated dislocations of the proximal radio-ulnar joint are not common but they should not be forgotten when examining films. In children the use of comparison views can be helpful, as in the case of this young gymnast (Figure 6.9). Here the left elbow is obviously abnormal when compared with the uninjured right elbow.

Because some fractures around the elbow can be easily missed, particularly supracondylar fractures in young children and radial head fractures in adults, the associated signs of a haemarthrosis should be looked for. The most useful of these is the presence of a displaced posterior fat pad which lies behind the distal end of the humerus as shown in Figure 6.10. If this sign is present, the bone should be carefully inspected and further views requested in an attempt to identify the occult fracture. In the illustration shown, which is a lateral of the elbow of a 28-year-old soccer player, there is a fracture of the radial head/neck but it is barely visible.

Another injury that is easily missed on X-ray is an avulsion of the medial epicondyle. In the example shown (Figure 6.11) of the left elbow of a young athlete, comparison views had been obtained which made the diagnosis much more straightforward. The avulsed epiphysis may be included within the elbow joint and if this injury is overlooked the long-term sequelae are serious. Less severe avulsions are even more difficult to diagnose and may require the use of oblique views as seen in Figure 6.12 which illustrates such an injury in a young weight-lifter.

Osteochondral fractures are often elusive although screening the suspected joint using fluoroscopy and image intensification may help to demonstrate the abnormality. As osteochondritis is also seen in the elbow joint, the usual sites being the capitulum and the radial head, it can be difficult to know whether one is dealing with an acute osteochondral fracture or osteochondritis. Osteochondritis may resolve completely or may result in loose bodies lying within the joint, as has occurred in this young tennis player (Figure 6.13). These loose bodies seem to flourish in the synovial fluid and can gradually increase in size as seen in Figures 6.14 and 6.15 which are views of the case illustrated in Figure 6.13. These films were taken at annual intervals over three years and, as can be seen, the intra-articular loose body has become quite sizeable and has led to recurrent pain and locking in the joint.

Repeated minor trauma may also result in multiple loose bodies within

Figure 6.2. Localized anteroposterior view of the head of the radius showing an undisplaced 'crack' fracture of the radial head.

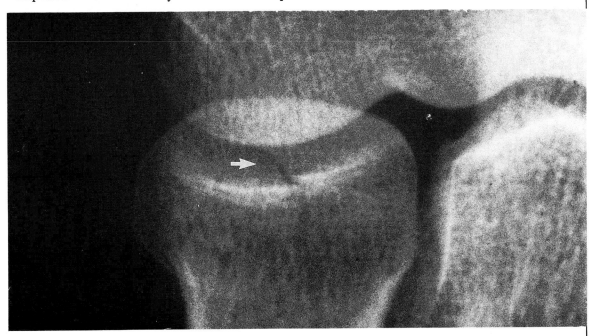

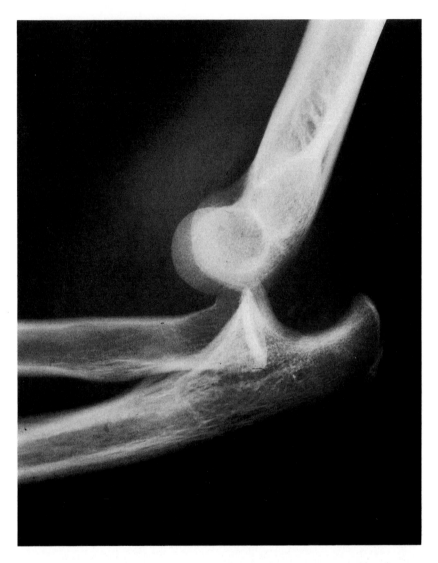

Figure 6.3. Lateral X-ray of an adult elbow showing a dislocation of the joint.

the joint as seen in Figure 6.16. This case occurred in an ex-javelin thrower and could easily be confused with synovial osteochondromatosis.

Soft tissue lesions around the elbow which are related to sporting activities are very common, for instance tennis elbow and golfer's elbow, and athletes whose events involve throwing or who play racquet sports will suffer damage to ligamentous and muscular insertions/origins around the joint. Occasionally there will be evidence of this on plain radiographs where small areas of calcification and ossification develop as in Figure 6.17 which illustrates this phenomenon in the ulnar collateral ligament. Xerography may be more sensitive than routine films and we occasionally use this technique to look for microcalcification. Repeated trauma to the elbow as seen in baseball pitchers leads to the typical 'Little Leaguer's elbow' (Figure 6.18), a significant problem for the adolescent athlete who is playing/practising a great deal.

The demonstration of radiolucent bodies within the elbow joint may be very difficult and the standard investigation is a single contrast arthrogram, using either contrast medium or air. Figure 6.19 shows an air arthrogram in a young gymnast with pain and a vague history of 'locking', although here no loose body was shown. Single contrast medium can also be used although it should be quite dilute or lucent bodies may be obscured. In Figure 6.20 a single contrast arthrogram has been performed in a young gymnast who previously sustained a severe injury. The arthrogram clearly shows that the radial head is displaced due to a fracture through the radial neck, and the fracture has united in an abnormal position. A combination of double contrast arthrography with or without CT will give yet more information, as it does in the shoulder joint. Scintigraphy is also occasionally useful in the demonstration of occult lesions as described in previous chapters, and MRI appears, from our short experience, to be a very promising investigation for soft tissue sporting injuries.

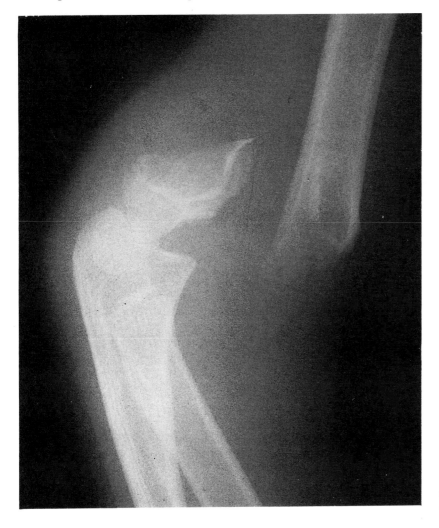

Figure 6.4. Lateral view of the elbow in a child showing a grossly displaced supracondylar fracture.

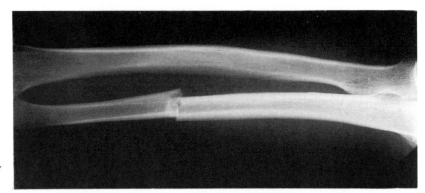

Figure 6.5. Anteroposterior view of the forearm showing an isolated middle third fracture of the ulna due to a direct blow.

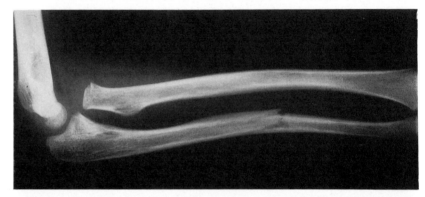

Figure 6.6. Angulated fracture of the middle third of the ulna. Note the associated anterior dislocation of the proximal end of the radius (Monteggia fracture).

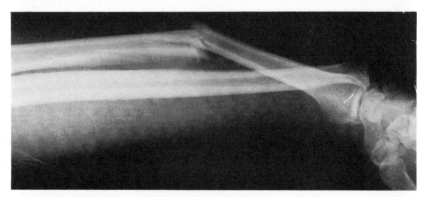

Figure 6.7. Angulated fracture of the distal third of the radius with an associated dislocation of the distal radio-ulnar joint (Galeazzi fracture).

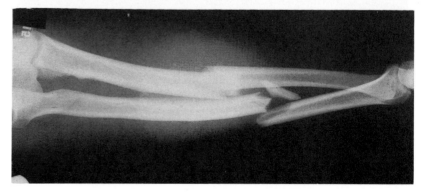

Figure 6.8. Mid-third fractures of the radius and ulna. Note the associated dislocation of the proximal end of the radius.

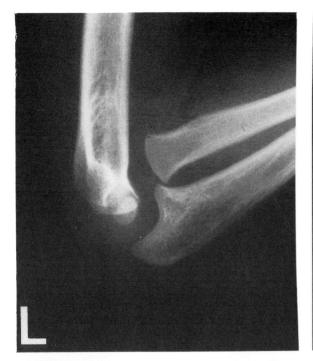

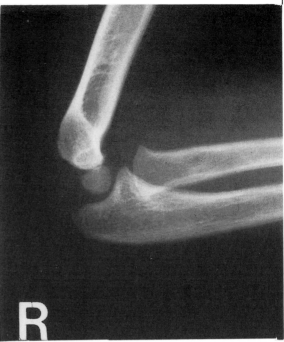

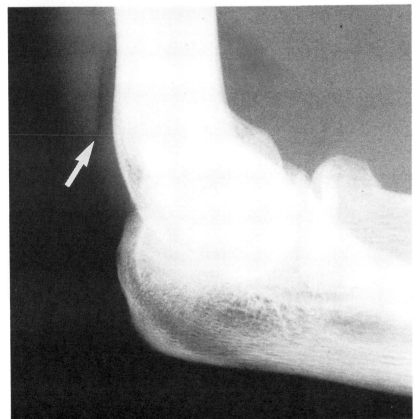

Figure 6.9. (Above). Lateral views of the elbows in a young gymnast. The right side is normal, but there is a dislocation of the left proximal radio-ulnar joint, the radius lying anteriorly.

Figure 6.10. (Left). Adult elbow, lateral view. Note the displaced posterior fat pad. Careful inspection shows a fracture of the radial head.

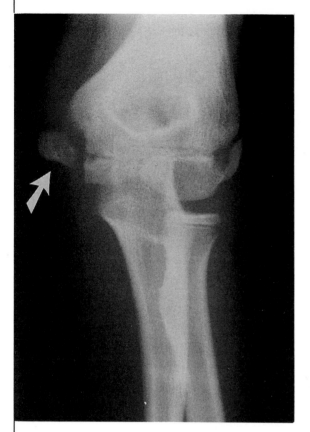

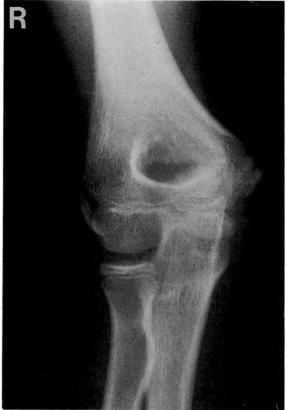

Figure 6.11. (Above). Anteroposterior views of the elbows in a young athlete. The right side is normal. The left side shows an avulsed medial epicondyle.

Figure 6.12. (Right). Localized anteroposterior view of the elbow demonstrating avulsion of the medial epicondyle (arrow).

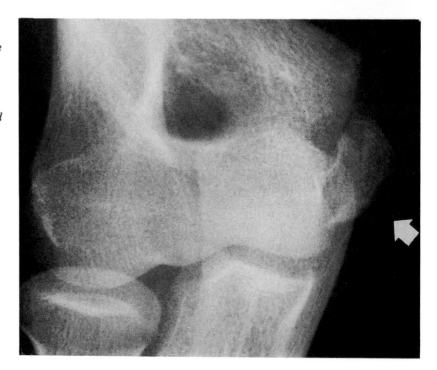

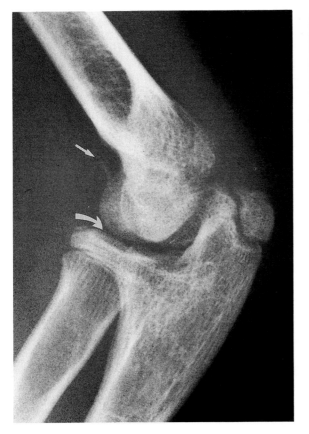

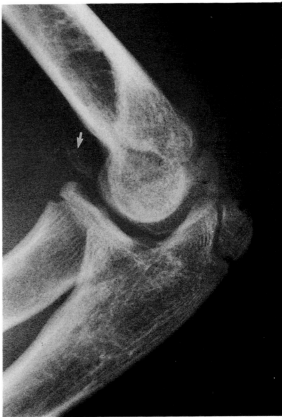

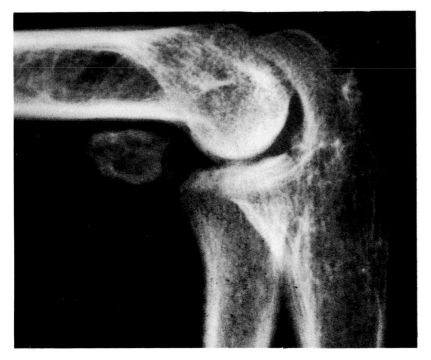

Figure 6.13. (Above left). Small intra-articular loose body (straight arrow). This is an osteochondral fragment which has arisen from the radial head (curved arrow).

Figure 6.14. (Above right). The same case as Figure 6.13 but some 12 months later. The osteochondral defect in the radial head and the loose body have increased in size.

Figure 6.15. (Left). The same case as Figures 6.13 and 6.14. The osteochondral fragment in the joint is now quite large.

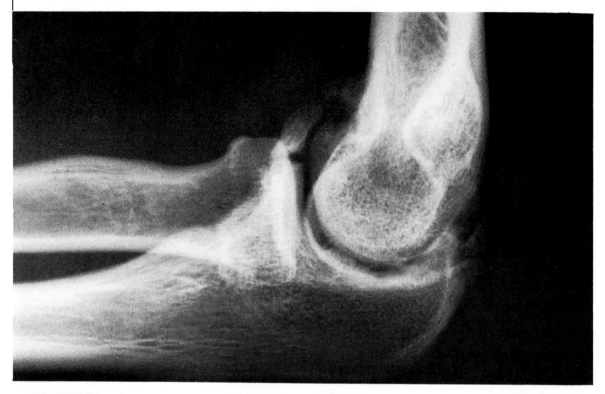

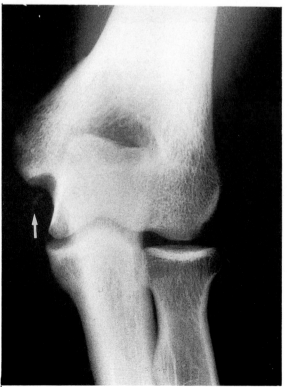

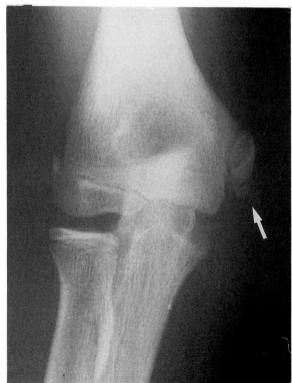

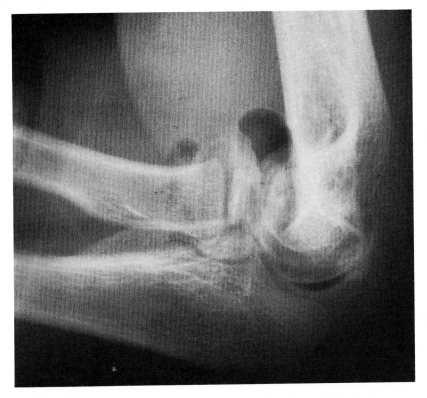

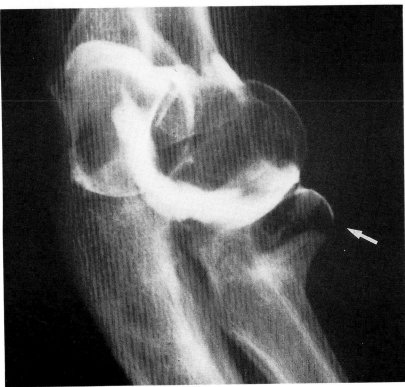

Figure 6.16. (Facing top).
Lateral X-ray of the elbow in
an adult who has sustained
multiple episodes of minor
trauma, showing numerous
small loose bodies.

Figure 6.17. (Facing bottom
left). Anteroposterior view of
the elbow in an adult. There is
some irregularity of the medial
epicondyle, and some calcified
areas below the medial
epicondyle due to repeated
strains on the joint ligaments
are faintly visible (arrow).

Figure 6.18. (Facing bottom
right). Anteroposterior X-ray of
the elbow of an adolescent
showing a very irregular
medial epicondyle due to over-
use injury in a young baseball
player.

Figure 6.19. Air arthrogram in
a young gymnast undertaken in
an attempt to demonstrate
radiolucent intra-articular loose
bodies. This examination is
normal.

Figure 6.20. Single contrast
arthrogram in a young
gymnast. There is a grossly
displaced radial head which has
fused to the shaft of the radius
in an abnormal position,
following a previous injury.

• BIBLIOGRAPHY •

Bede, W. B., Lefebure, A. R. and Roseman, M. A. (1975) Fractures of the medial humeral epicondyle in children. *Can. J. Surg.* **18**, 137.

Bell, R. H. and Hawkins, R. J. (1986) Stress fracture of the distal ulna. *Clin. Orthop.* **209**, 169.

Borris, L. C., Lassen, M. R. and Christensen, C. S. (1987) Elbow dislocation in children and adults. *Acta Orthop. Scand.* **58**, 649.

Brogdon, B. G. and Crops, N. W. (1960) Little Leaguer's elbow. *Am. J. Radiol.* **83**, 671.

Brown, R., Blazina, M. E., Kerlan, R. K., *et al.* (1974) Osteochondritis of the capitulum. *Am. J. Sports Med.* **2**, 27.

Bruce, H. E., Harvey, J. P. and Wilson, J. C. (1974) Monteggia fractures. *J. Bone Joint Surg.* **56(A)**, 1563.

Buhl, O. and Hellberg, S. (1982) Displaced supracondylar fractures of the humerus in children. *Acta Orthop. Scand.* **53**, 67.

Chessare, J. W., Rogers, L. F., White, H., *et al.* (1977) Injuries of the medial epicondylar ossification centre of the humerus. *Am. J. Radiol.* **129**, 49.

Colton, C. L. (1973) Fractures of the olecranon in adults: classification and management. *Injury* **5**, 121.

Conn, J. Jr. and Wade, P. A. (1961) Injuries of the elbow: a ten year review. *J. Trauma* **1**, 248.

Dehaven, K. E. and Evarts, C. M. (1973) Throwing injuries of the elbow in athletes. *Orthop. Clin. N. Am.* **4**, 801.

Eto, R. T., Anderson, P. W. and Harley, J. D. (1975) Elbow arthrography with the application of tomography. *Radiology* **115**, 283.

Gore, R. M., Rogers, L. F., Bowerman, J., *et al.* (1980) Osseous manifestations of elbow stress associated with sports activities. *Am. J. Radiol.* **134**, 971.

Greenspan, A. and Norman, A. (1987) Radial head-capitellum view: an expanded imaging approach to elbow injury. *Radiology* **164**, 272.

Gugenheim, J. J., Stanley, R. F., Woods, G. W., *et al.* (1976) Little League survey: the Houston study. *Am. J. Sports Med.* **4**, 189.

Guistra, P. E., Killoran, P. J., Furman, R. S. and Root, J. A. (1974) Missed Monteggia fracture. *Radiology* **110**, 45.

Hall-Craggs, M. A., Shorvon, P. J. and Chapman, M. (1985) Assessment of the radial head-capitellum view and the dorsal fat-pad sign in acute elbow trauma. *Am. J. Radiol.* **145**, 607.

Hamilton, H. K. (1984) Stress fracture of the diaphysis of the ulna in a body builder. *Am. J. Sports Med.* **12(5)**, 105.

Hendrikson, B. (1966) Supracondylar fracture of the humerus in children. *Acta Chir. Scand.* Supplementum **369**, 1.

Horne, J. G. and Tanzer, T. L. (1981) Olecranon fractures: a review of 100 cases. *J. Trauma* **21**, 469.

Hudson, T. M. (1984) Joint fluoroscopy before arthrography: detection and evaluation of loose bodies. *Skeletal Radiol.* **12**, 199.

Johansson, O. (1962) Capsular and ligament injuries of the elbow joint: a clinical and arthrographic study. *Acta. Chir. Scand.* Supplementum **287**, 5.

Josefesson, P. O., Johnell, O. and Gentz, C. F. (1984) Long-term sequelae of simple dislocation of the elbow. *J. Bone Joint Surg.* **66(A)**, 927.

King, J. W., Brelsford, H. J. and Tullos, H. S. (1969) Analysis of the pitching arm of the professional baseball pitcher. *Clin. Orthop.* **67**, 116.

Kramhoft, M. D., Keller, I. L. and Solgaard, S. M. D. (1987) Displaced supracondylar fractures of the humerus in children. *Clin. Orthop.* **221**, 215.

Mann, T. S. (1963) Prognosis in supracondylar fractures. *J. Bone Joint Surg.* **45(B)**, 516.

Mehloff, T. L., Noble, P. C., Bennett, J. B. and Tullos, H. S. (1988) Simple dislocation of the elbow in the adult. *J. Bone Joint Surg.* **70(A)**, 244.

Micheli, L. J. (1983) Overuse injuries in children's sports: the growth factor. *Orthop. Clin. N. Am.* **14(2)**, 337.

Miklic, Z. D. (1975) Galeazzi fracture-dislocations. *J. Bone Joint Surg.* **57(A)**, 1071.

Miller, J. E. (1960) Javelin thrower's elbow. *J. Bone Joint Surg.* **42(B)**, 788.

Mino, D. E., Palmer, A. K. and Levinsohn, E. M. (1983) The role of radiography and computerised tomography in the diagnosis of subluxation and dislocation of the distal radioulnar joint. *J. Hand Surg.* **8**, 23.

Mitsunaga, M. M., Adishian, D. A. and Bianco, A. J. (1982) Osteochondritis dissecans of the capitellum. *J. Trauma* **22(1)**, 53.

Morrey, B. F. and An, K. N. (1983) Articular and ligamentous contributions to the stability of the elbow joint. *Am. J. Sports Med.* **11**, 315.

Morrey, B. F., An, K. N. and Stormont, T. J.

(1988) Force transmission through the radial head. *J. Bone Joint Surg.* **70(A)**, 250.

Murphy, W. A. and Siegel, M. J. (1977) Elbow fat-pads with new signs and extended differential diagnosis. *Radiology* **124**, 659.

Mutoh, Y., Mori, T., Suzuki, Y., *et al.* (1982) Stress fractures of the ulna in athletes. *Am. J. Sports Med.* **10(6)**, 365.

Neviaser, J. S. and Wickstrom, J. K. (1977) Dislocation of the elbow: a retrospective study of 115 patients. *Southern Med. J.* **70**, 172.

Nirschl, R. P. and Pettrone, F. A. (1979) Tennis elbow. *J. Bone Joint Surg.* **61(A)**, 832.

Palmer, E. E., Niemann, K. M. W., Vesely, D. and Armstrong, J. H. (1978) Supracondylar fracture of the humerus in children. *J. Bone Joint Surg.* **60(A)**, 653.

Papavasilious, V. A. (1982) Fracture-separation of the medial epicondylar epiphysis of the elbow joint. *Clin. Orthop.* **171**, 172.

Pappas, A. M. (1982) Elbow problems associated with baseball during childhood and adolescence. *Clin. Orthop.* **164**, 30.

Pavlov, H., Ghelman, B. and Warren, R. F. (1979) Double contrast arthrography of the elbow. *Radiology* **130**, 87.

Peiro, A., Andres, F. and Fernandez-Esteve, F. (1977) Acute Monteggia lesions in children. *J. Bone Joint Surg.* **59(A)**, 92.

Piggot, J. A., Graham, H. K. and McCoy, G. F. (1986) Supracondylar fractures of the humerus in children. *J. Bone Joint Surg.* **68(B)**, 577.

Poulsen, J. O. and Tophoj, K. (1974) Fracture of the head and neck of the radius. *Acta Orthop. Scand.* **45**, 66.

Priest, J. D., Broden, V. M. A. and Gerberick, J. G. (1980) The elbow and tennis. Part I: An analysis of players with and without pain. *Phys. Sports Med.* **9(4)**, 80.

Quinton, D. N., Finlay, D. and Butterworth, R. (1987) The elbow fat-pad sign. *J. Bone Joint Surg.* **69(B)**, 844.

Reckling, F. W. (1982) Unstable fracture-dislocations of the forearm (Monteggia and Galeazzi lesions). *J. Bone Joint Surg.* **64(A)**, 857.

Rettig, A. C. (1983) Stress fracture of the ulna in an adolescent tournament tennis player. *Am. J. Sports Med.* **11(2)**, 103.

Singer, K. M. and Roy, S. P. (1984) Osteochondrosis of the humeral capitellum. *Am. J. Sports Med.* **12**, 351.

Smith, F. M. (1950) Medial epicondyle injuries: *J. Am. Med. Ass.* **142**, 396.

Tullos, H. S. and King, J. W. (1972) Lesions of the pitching arm in adolescents. *J. Am. Med. Ass.* **220**, 264.

Tullos, H. S. and King, J. W. (1973) Throwing mechanism in sports. *Orthop. Clin. N. Am.* **4**, 709.

Walsh, H. P. J., McLaren, C. A. N. and Owen, R. (1987) Galeazzi fractures in children. *J. Bone Joint Surg.* **69(B)**, 730.

Wojtys, E. M. (1987) Sports injuries in the immature athlete. *Orthop. Clin. N. Am.* **18**, 689.

Woods, G. W. and Tullos, H. S. (1977) Elbow instability and medial epicondyle fractures. *Am. J. Sports Med.* **5**, 23.

Woods, G. W., Tullos, H. S. and King, J. W. (1973) The throwing arm: elbow joint injuries. *Am. J. Sports Med.* **1**, 43.

Woodward, A. H. and Bianco, A. J. Jr. (1975) Osteochondritis dissecans of the elbow. *Clin. Orthop.* **110**, 35.

Zarins, B., Andrews, J. R. and Carson, W. (1985) Injuries of the throwing arm. Philadelphia: W. B. Saunders.

7 The Wrist and Hand

Fractures and dislocations of the bones of the wrist and hand are a common consequence of contact sports as well as 'hand ball' games, such as volleyball, basketball and netball, and certain of the 'hard ball' games, such as baseball and cricket.

Damage to the carpal bones is rare in children while people aged over 40 years who fall onto their outstretched hand usually sustain a Colles' fracture. However, young adults, the group most commonly engaged in sporting activities, are the ones most likely to sustain fractures of the carpals (most frequently the scaphoid bone) and dislocations in the area.

Injuries such as a fractured scaphoid can be difficult to diagnose; plain films may initially be passed as normal, although many of these fractures are detectable if looked for closely enough. However, if the investigation is repeated after two weeks or so, changes will have become visible (Figure 7.1) due to slight resorption of bone around the previously undetectable fracture line. Figure 7.1 is the plain film of the right wrist of a 21-year-old rugby player who has sustained an injury some six weeks previously and in whom the scaphoid fracture is now clearly visible. Where symptoms persist, and later films are still undiagnostic, an isotope bone scan is the investigation of choice. Figure 7.2 shows a positive scan demonstrating a fractured scaphoid in the left wrist of a 20-year-old tennis player whose plain films were unremarkable. Had the scan been normal at this stage (two weeks after the incident) the chances of a fracture being present would have been remote. The problem of delayed union, or non-union or ischaemic necrosis of the proximal half of the scaphoid is a serious one, particularly in athletes who are active in the racquet sports.

Dislocations of the carpal bones are uncommon and, perhaps because of this, are easily missed on X-ray. Violent hyperextension injuries of the wrist may result in a lunate dislocation, the bone typically dislocating into the palmar surface of the joint. This is best appreciated on the lateral film as shown in Figure 7.3 which is a view of the left wrist of a 24-year-old soccer player who fell onto his outstretched left hand.

As in other areas of the musculoskeletal system, the most difficult problem is a symptomatic patient who has no diagnostic clinical signs and whose radiographs are normal. Under these circumstances, isotope bone scanning is an excellent screening test. Figure 7.4 shows a bone scan of the wrist and hands of a golfer complaining of pain in the right wrist. The scan is diffusely hot, an appearance that can in fact result from disuse. However, this guided the radiologist to further investigation (CT scanning) which revealed in Figure 7.5 a fracture of the hook of the hamate bone. These fractures occur in baseball players, golfers and those who engage in racquet sports where the handle violently strikes the palmar surface of the wrist. While the injury may be suspected from the clinical history, even specialized carpal tunnel views (Figure 7.6 as in this 28-year-old baseball player may not demonstrate a fracture. However, a bone scan performed two or three days later (Figure 7.7) revealed a focal area of increased uptake in the hamate. The investigation of choice at present is probably a CT scan; however, care must be taken in the interpretation of the film because, if the slices are not right through the base of the hook, an apparent 'fracture' may be demonstrated. Where views are equivocal, scanning of both wrists may be necessary for comparison purposes.

Figure 7.1. Oblique view of the right wrist demonstrating the scaphoid. There is an un-united fracture (arrow) showing resorption around the fracture line with some sclerosis. The injury was sustained six weeks before this film was taken.

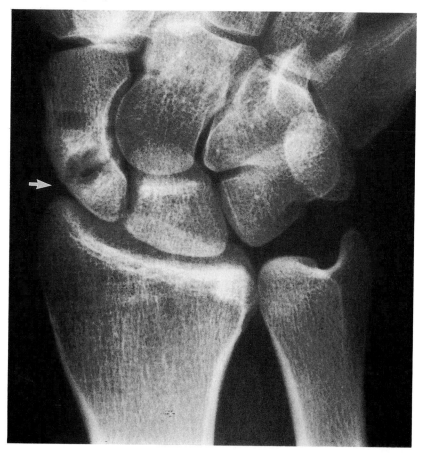

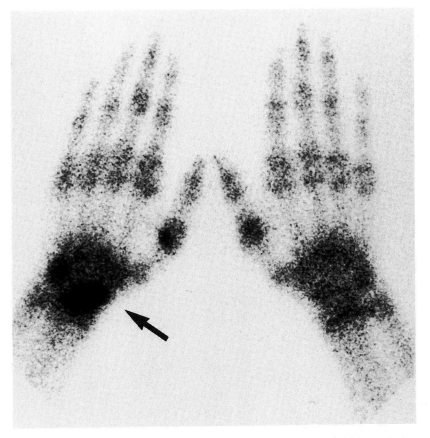

Figure 7.2. Bone scan of the wrists/hands of a young man with 'normal' X-rays. This shows an area of increased uptake in the left wrist compared with the right, particularly in the region of the scaphoid (arrow). The appearances are due to increased bony activity in the scaphoid from a previously undiagnosed fracture. The general 'background' activity is due to disuse.

The metacarpal bone most commonly fractured is the fifth, and the usual site of injury is the neck of the bone. Figure 7.8 illustrates such a 'punch' injury in the hand of a 27-year-old rugby player. The fracture was clinically obvious due to the deformity produced and was treated conservatively with short-term garter strapping and subsequent mobilization.

Oblique fractures of other metacarpals occur quite frequently and are usually managed conservatively with a good result. One of the more serious injuries, however, is that to the base of the first metacarpal, the so-called Bennett's fracture dislocation/subluxation. Fractures of the base of the first metacarpal uncomplicated by dislocation/subluxation occur classically in boxing, and Figure 7.9 illustrates a displaced fracture at the base of the first metacarpal in a 19-year-old boxer which subsequently required reduction and stabilization.

The first metacarpophalangeal joint is also prone to injuries in relation to its collateral ligaments, usually resulting from hyperextension injuries. If the tear is complete, instability results and surgical repair may be indicated shortly after the injury. Such damage may be diagnosed (Figure 7.10) where there is an avulsed fragment as in this 30-year-old skier, an injury that was sustained on a dry ski-slope. In view of the frequency of such injuries in this particular sport it has been identified as 'skier's'

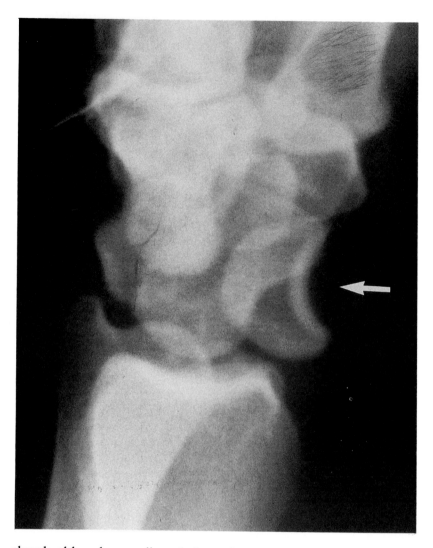

Figure 7.3. Lateral X-ray of a wrist showing a dislocated lunate (arrow).

thumb, although more distantly it was known as 'gamekeeper's' thumb. Avulsed fragments may become quite large as illustrated in Figure 7.11 which is an X-ray of the thumb of a 26-year-old cricketer whose injury had occurred 12 months previously. Stress views (Figure 7.12) demonstrate some instability at the first metacarpophalangeal joint, although at this stage it was not felt that surgical intervention would be helpful to his sporting career.

Damage to the radial collateral ligament is seen only rarely although, as shown in Figure 7.13, it can occur and give rise to similar problems. This injury was sustained by a 23-year-old basketball player.

The hard ball used in sports such as baseball, cricket and hockey inevitably produces damage to the hands when participants are struck by a flying ball or even by the stick itself. Figure 7.14 shows the hand of a 26-year-old field hockey player who sustained a blow forceful enough to fracture the proximal phalanx of her little finger.

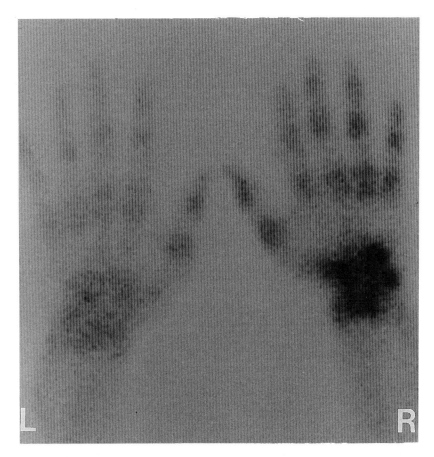

Figure 7.4. Bone scan of hands/wrists showing generalized disuse activity in the right wrist but with no convincing focal 'hot spot'.

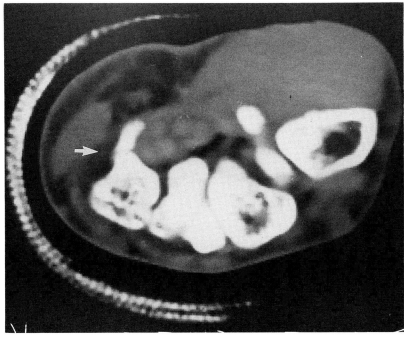

Figure 7.5. CT scan of the wrist showing a fracture of the base of the hook of the hamate.

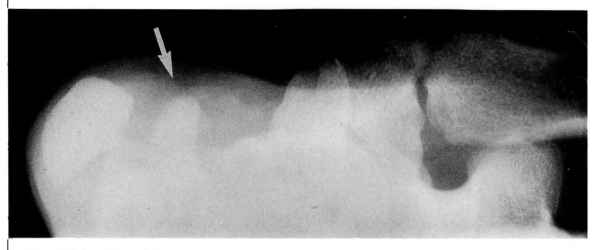

Figure 7.6. Carpal tunnel view showing a 'normal' hook of hamate.

Fractures of the phalanges are often disregarded but they should not be treated lightly as they may lead to long-term disability due to deformity and tethering of tendons. Fractures involving the interphalangeal joints almost invariably lead to permanently swollen joints which have a reduced range of movement.

The typical mallet finger deformity occurs when an athlete attempting to catch or parry a ball is struck on the end of the finger and the distal interphalangeal joint is hyperflexed. The injury illustrated in Figure 7.15 occurred to a 21-year-old goalkeeper, and eventually a hand surgeon had to fuse the two phalanges (Figure 7.16) in order to allow him to continue with his career.

Injuries affecting the volar plate are serious, and subsequent suboptimal function of the hand is a common permanent sequel. Such injuries may well produce negative radiographs, although this is not the case where there is an associated avulsion as in the lateral view of the middle finger (Figure 7.17) of this 23-year-old basketball player.

Figure 7.18 illustrates a particularly severe injury of this type with disruption of the flexor and extensor mechanisms of the finger and associated ligamentous damage to the proximal interphalangeal joint. This was sustained by a 34-year-old cricketer and effectively ended his participation in the sport.

Hand injuries in boxers can also dramatically retard or even end their careers in the ring, and the punishment sustained by the bones in the wrist and hand when working out on the heavy bag or when actually fighting is considerable. Complaints of pain in the hand/wrist are common and, although plain X-rays are usually normal, a bone scan often demonstrates the stresses imposed upon these structures. Figure 7.19 shows the hands of an orthodox (right-handed) middle-weight boxer. The right hand, the one with which his heaviest punch is landed, is significantly 'hotter' than the left. Similar changes may be found in the hands of some exponents of the martial arts, particularly full contact karate and those who indulge in 'breaking'.

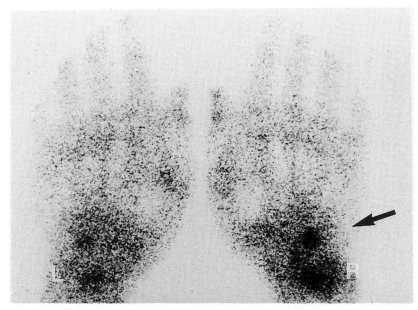

Figure 7.7. Bone scan of the wrists/hands showing increased activity on the right side. There are two localized 'hot spots', one in the region of the radio-ulnar joint and the other at the hamate (arrow).

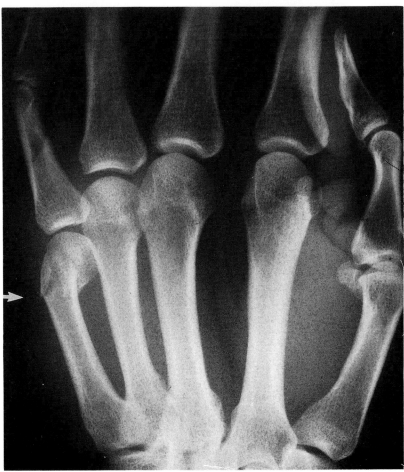

Figure 7.8. Angulated fracture of the neck of the fifth metacarpal of the left hand (arrow) producing shortening and loss of the normal 'knuckle'.

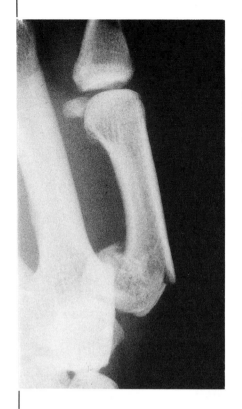

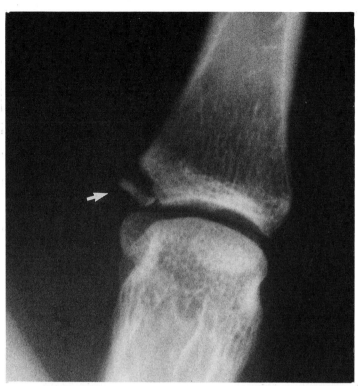

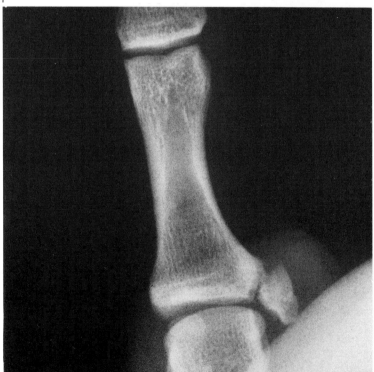

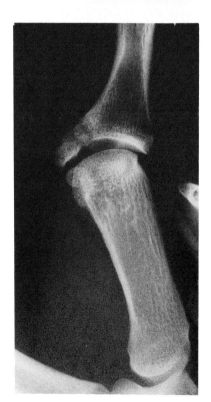

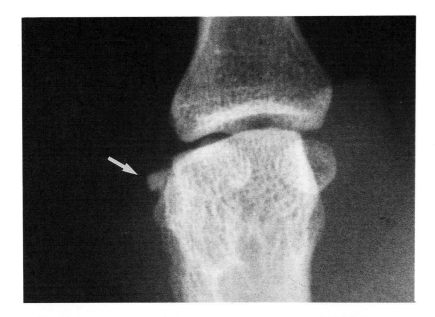

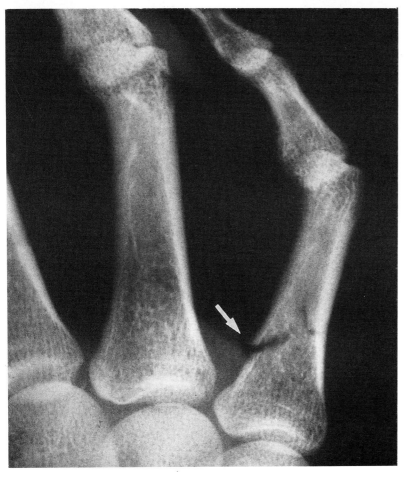

Figure 7.9. (Facing top left). Displaced fracture at the base of the first metacarpal sustained by a boxer.

Figure 7.10. (facing top right). Localized view of the first metacarpophalangeal joint showing a small avulsion fragment secondary to damage to the ulnar collateral ligament (skier's/gamekeeper's thumb).

Figure 7.11. (Facing bottom left). Pseudoarthrosis of the base of the proximal phalanx of the thumb due to a chronic ulnar collateral injury.

Figure 7.12. (Facing bottom right). Stressed view of skier's/gamekeeper's thumb demonstrating some instability.

Figure 7.13. (Above left). Localized view of the first metacarpophalangeal joint showing normal sesamoid bones but also a small avulsion on the radial side of the first metacarpal, indicating damage to the radial collateral ligament.

Figure 7.14. (Left). Oblique fracture of the proximal phalanx of the little finger of a left hand.

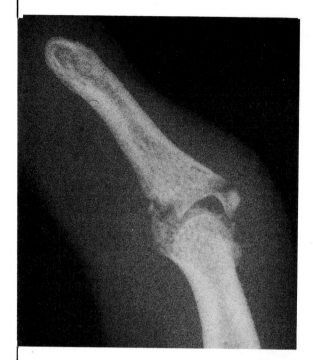

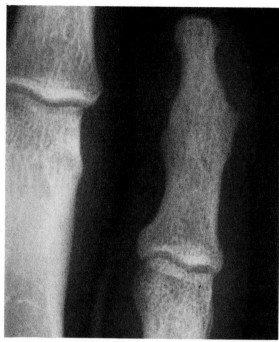

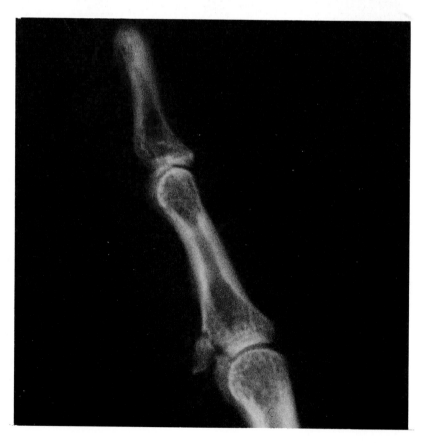

Figure 7.15. (Above left). Lateral view of the distal interphalangeal joint of the little finger of the right hand showing a typical mallet finger deformity.

Figure 7.16. (Above right). Anteroposterior view of the little finger (same case as Figure 7.15) showing complete ankylosis of the distal interphalangeal joint.

Figure 7.17. (Right). Lateral joint of finger with a typical volar plate injury at the base of the middle phalanx involving the proximal interphalangeal joint.

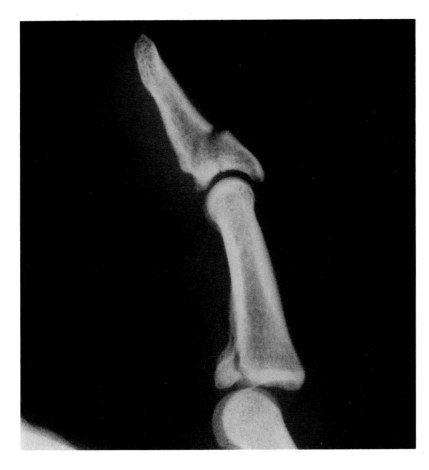

Figure 7.18. (Left). Lateral view of the finger of a netball player with a fracture at the terminal phalanx involving the distal interphalangeal joint, and also a volar plate injury at the base of the middle phalanx with dorsal subluxation of the proximal interphalangeal joint.

Figure 7.19. (Below). Bone scan of the hands of a middle-weight boxer who was an orthodox (right-handed) puncher. The scans show increased activity in both wrists and interphalangeal joints, but more particularly on the right.

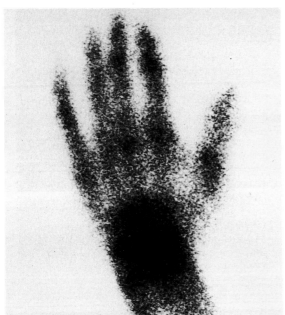
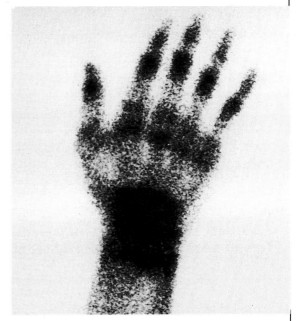

● BIBLIOGRAPHY ●

Belsole, R. J., Eikman, E. A., and Muroff, L. R. (1981) Bone scintigraphy in trauma of the hand and wrist. *J. Trauma* **21**, 163.

Bennett, E. H. (1886) On fracture of the metacarpal bone of the thumb. *Br. Med. J.* **2**, 12.

Blitzer, C. M., Johnson, R. J., Ettlinger, C. F. and Aggeborn, K. (1984) Downhill skiing injuries in children. *Am. J. Sports Med.* **12**, 142.

Borgeskove, S., Christiansen, B., Kjaer, A. and Balslev, I. (1966) Fracture of the carpal bones. *Acta Orth. Scand.* **37**, 276.

Bowers, W. and Hurst, L. (1977) Gamekeeper's thumb. *J. Bone Joint Surg.* **59(A)**, 514.

Bowers, W. H. and Hurst, L. C. (1977) Gamekeeper's thumb. Evaluation by arthrography and stress roentgenography. *J. Bone Joint Surg.* **59(A)**, 519.

Browne, E. J. Jr., Dunn, H. K. and Snyder, C. C. (1976) Ski pole thumb injury. *Plast. Reconstr. Surg.* **68**, 19.

Burke, F. D. (1988) Mallet finger. *J. Hand Surg.* **13(B)**, 115.

Burton, R. I. and Eaton, R. G. (1973) Common hand injuries in the athlete. *Orthop. Clin. N. Am.* **4**, 809.

Campbell, C. (1955) Gamekeeper's thumb. *J. Bone Joint Surg.* **37(B)**, 148.

Campbell, R. D., Lance, E. M. and Yeoh, C. B. (1964) Lunate and perilunar dislocations. *J. Bone Joint Surg.* **46(B)**, 55.

Carr, D., Johnson, R. and Pope, M. (1981) Upper extremity injuries in skiing. *Am. J. Sports Med.* **9**, 378.

Carter, R., Eaton, R. G. and Littler, J. W. (1977) Ununited fracture of the hook of the hamate. *J. Bone Joint Surg.* **59(A)**, 583.

Collins, R. K. (1987) Injury patterns in women's intra-mural flag football. *Am. J. Sports Med.* **15**, 238.

Curtin J. and Kay, N. R. M. (1976) Hand injuries due to soccer. *The Hand* **8**, 93.

Dacruz, D. J., Bodiwala, G. G. and Finlay, D. B. L. (1988) The suspected fracture of the scaphoid: a rational approach to diagnosis. *Injury* **19(3)**, 149.

Davidson, R. M. (1987) Schoolboy rugby injuries. *Med. J. Austr.* **147**, 119.

Destot, E. (1986) Injuries to the wrist. *Clin. Orthop.* **202**, 3.

Deyerle, W. M. (1962) Athletic injuries of the upper extremities. *Clin. Orthop.* **23**, 84.

Dobyns, J. H. and Linscheid, R. L. (1980) Carpal bone injuries. *Clin. Orthop.* **149**, 2.

Dobyns, J. H., Sim, F. H. and Linscheid, R. L. (1978) Sports stress syndromes of the hand and wrist. *Am. J. Sports Med.* **6**, 236.

Downey, E. F. and Curtis, D. J. (1986) Patient-induced stress test of the first metacarpophalangeal joint: a radiographic assessment of collateral ligament injuries. *Radiology* **158**, 679.

Ellasser, J. C. and Stein, A. H. (1979) Management of hand injuries in a professional football team. *Am. J. Sports Med.* **7**, 178.

Fisk, G. R. (1981) An overview of injuries of the wrist. *Clin. Orthop.* **149**, 137.

Flatt, A. E. (1967) Athletic injuries of the hand. *J. Louis. State Med. Soc.* **119**, 425.

Ganel, A., Engel, J., Oster, Z., *et al.* (1979) Bone scanning in assessment of fractures of the scaphoid. *J. Hand Surg.* **4**, 540.

Gerber, C., Senn, E. and Matter, P. (1981) Skier's thumb. *Am. J. Sports Med.* **9**, 171.

Goldberg, B. *et al.* (1988) Injuries in youth football. *Paediatrics* **81(2)**, 255.

Helm, R. H. (1987) Hand function after injuries to the collateral ligaments of the metacarpophalangeal joint of the thumb. *J. Hand Surg.* **12(B)**, 252.

Inkelis, S. H., Stroberg, A. J., Keller, E. L. and Christenson, P. D. (1988) Roller skating injuries in children. *Paed. Em. Care* **4(2)**, 127.

Jorgensen, T. M., Andreson, J. H., Thommesen, P., *et al.* (1979) Scanning and radiology of the carpal scaphoid bone. *Acta Ortho. Scand.* **50**, 663.

Kessler, I. (1963) Complete avulsion of the ulnar collateral ligament of the metacarpophalangeal joint of the thumb. *Clin. Orthop.* **29**, 196.

Kleinert, J. M. and Zenni, E. J. (1984) Nonunion of the scaphoid: review of the literature and current treatment. *Orthop. Rev.* **13**, 125.'

Leddy, J. P. and Packer, J. W. (1977) Avulsion of the profundus insertion in athletes. *J. Hand Surg.* **2**, 66.

Linscheid, R. L. and Dobyns, J. H. (1985) Athletic injuries of the wrist. *Clin. Orthop.* **198**, 141.

McCue, F. C., Honner, R., Johnson, M. and Gieck, J. H. (1970) Athletic injuries of the proximal interphalangeal joint requiring surgical treatment. *J. Bone Joint Surg.* **52(A)**, 937.

McCue, F. C., Andrews, J. R. and Hakala, N. W. (1974) The coach's finger. *Am. J. Sports Med.* **2**, 270.

McCue, F. C., Hakala, M. W., Andrews, J. R. and Gieck, J. H. (1974) Ulnar collateral ligament injuries of the thumb in athletes. *J. Sports Med.* **2**, 70.

McCue, F. C., Baugher, W. H., Kulund, D. N. and Gieck, J. H. (1978) Hand and wrist injuries in the athlete. *Am. J. Sports Med.* **7**, 275.

Mack, G. R., Bosse, M. J., Gelberman, R. H. and Yu, E. (1984) The natural history of scaphoid nonunion. *J. Bone Joint Surg.* **66(A)**, 504.

Mayfield, J. K., Johnson, R. P. and Kilcoyne, R. K. (1980) Carpal dislocations: pathomechanics and progressive perilunar instability. *J. Hand Surg.* **5**, 226.

Neviaser, R. J., Wilson, J. N. and Lievano, A. (1971) Rupture of the ulnar collateral ligament of the thumb (Gamekeeper's thumb). Correction by dynamic repair. *J. Bone Joint Surg.* **53(A)**, 1357.

Palmer, A. K. and Louis, D. S. (1978) Assessing ulnar instability of the metacarpophalangeal joint of the thumb. *J. Hand Surg.* **3**, 542.

Parker, R. D., Berkowitz, M. S., Brahms, M. A., *et al.* (1986) Hook of the hamate fractures in athletes. *Am. J. Sports Med.* **14**, 517.

Sakellarides, H. (1978) Treatment of recent and old injuries of the ulnar collateral ligament of the MP joint of the thumb. *Am. J. Sports Med.* **6**, 255.

Smith, R. (1977) Post-traumatic instability of metacarpophalangeal joint of the thumb. *J. Bone Joint Surg.* **59(A)**, 14.

Stark, H. H., Jobe, F. W., Boyes, J. H. and Ashworth, C. R. (1977) Fracture of the hook of the hamate in athletes. *J. Bone Joint Surg.* **59(A)**, 575.

Steedman, D. J. (1986) Artificial ski slope injuries: a one-year prospective study. *Injury* **17**, 208.

Stordahl, A., Schjoth, A., Woxholf, G., *et al.* (1984) Bone scanning of fracture of the scaphoid. *J. Hand Surg.* **9(B)**, 189.

Sy, W. M., Bay, R. and Cameron, A. (1977) Hand images: normal and abnormal. *J. Nucl. Med.* **18**, 419.

Torisu, T. (1972) Fracture of the hook of the hamate by golfswing. *Clin. Orthop.* **83**, 91.

Watson, H. K. and Ballet, F. L. (1984) The SLAC wrist: scapholunate advanced collapse pattern of degenerative arthritis. *J. Hand Surg.* **9(A)**, 358.

Weller, S. (1961) Die Distorsion im Daumengrundgelenk als Skitrauma. *Dtsch. Med. Wochenschr.* **86**, 521.

Young, M. R. A., Lowry, J. H., Laird, J. D. and Ferguson, W. R. (1988) $^{99}Tc^{m}$-MDP bone scanning of injuries of the carpal scaphoid. *Injury* **19**, 14.

8 The Pelvis

Most injuries to the pelvis that we deal with are those to the muscular insertions in the area, and bony involvement is limited to tiny fragments that have sometimes been avulsed.

Fractures produced by direct violence to the structure are uncommon and usually occur in the motorized sports using all-terrain vehicles, or in high-risk or high-speed activities such as hang-gliding and downhill skiing.

As far as bony problems are concerned, stress injuries to the pelvic region are seen more commonly in our practice. Some of these may produce diagnostic plain films, but we frequently perform isotope bone scans where the ordinary radiographs are 'normal'. Triple phase scanning (TPS) is usually undertaken, the initial scan being done shortly after injection of the isotope and the second scan within a few minutes of the first. These two scans highlight any abnormal hyperaemia in the area and the stress fractures, if present, will be demonstrated by the third scan taken one to three hours later.

Figure 8.1 illustrates stress fractures that have occurred bilaterally in the femora of a long-distance runner. These were detectable on plain radiographs and are unusual in our experience as they occur in the femoral shaft. More commonly the stress fractures we see are found in the neck of the femur as illustrated in the bone scan (Figure 8.2) of a postmenopausal female jogger. Alternatively they are seen in the pubic rami, and Figure 8.3 shows such a lesion in a marathon runner, also a woman. Occasionally such fractures in the femoral neck come to surgical fixation but we attempt to avoid this wherever possible.

Pain in the region of the groin and the symphysis pubis is seen fairly frequently in both rugby and soccer players; it is often due to musculotendinous strains, and occasionally is related to osteitis pubis. This latter is a chronic problem produced by the stresses placed on the symphysis by the patient's sporting activity and it should not be confused with the inflammatory process sometimes seen in men with prostatic disease. Plain films are often diagnostic as in Figure 8.4, a localized view of the symphysis in a 29-year-old rugby forward, showing sclerosis and cyst formation together with erosions and osteophytes. The discomfort caused by this condition can be considerable and even with enthusiastic treatment patients can be out of their sports for many months. Instability of the symphysis is sometimes associated, and can be demonstrated by separate views taken with the patient standing on a single leg alternately (Flamingo views). Mild instability is demonstrated in Figure 8.5 which shows two views of the symphysis in a 23-year-old cricketer (a fast bowler).

Repeated sudden muscular contractures, particularly in the young skeleton, may result in the avulsion of bony fragments at the site of muscle origins/insertions. Figure 8.6 shows an avulsion of the anterior inferior iliac spine in a 14-year-old judo enthusiast, presumably caused by the pull of rectus femoris on its origin. The ischial tuberosity and lesser trochanter complex are also commonly involved in these injuries, and Figures 8.7 and 8.8 show an avulsion of the lesser trochanter on the right femur in a young hurdler.

The majority of such problems settle with conservative management

Figure 8.1. Periosteal reactions in both femora due, in this instance, to bilateral femoral shaft stress fractures.

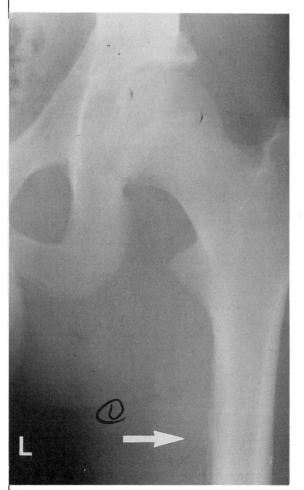

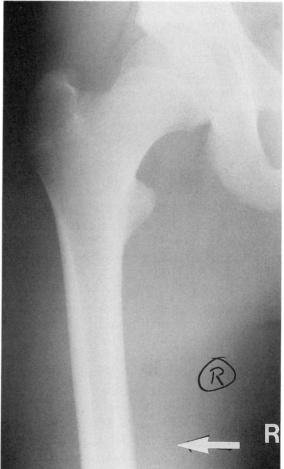

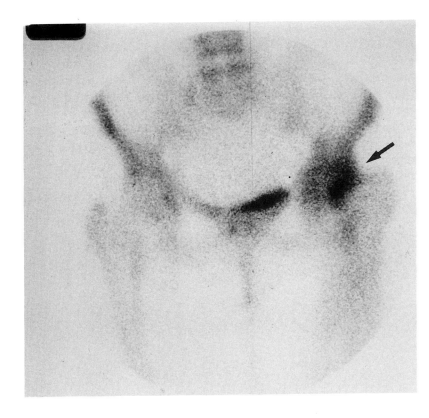

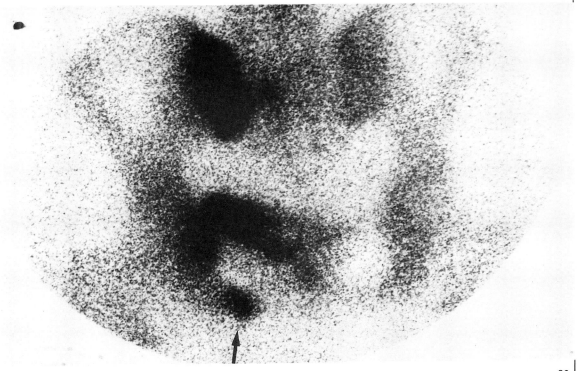

Figure 8.2. (Left). Isotope bone scan of the pelvis and hips. Note the area of activity in the bladder and also in the left femoral neck (arrow) due to a stress fracture.

Figure 8.3. (Below). Isotope bone scan of the pelvis showing abnormal activity in the pubic rami due to a stress fracture (arrow) and also increased activity in the sacroiliac region due to the extra stresses that have been placed upon the joint. Note also the activity in the bladder.

and do no more than temporarily impede the athlete's sporting career, even if larger fragments (Figure 8.9) are pulled off as is shown in the view of this young sprinter's pelvis: the whole of the ischial tuberosity has avulsed and gone on to formal non-union. This is also the case in Figure 8.10 where there is a large avulsed fragment still obviously separated in a 27-year-old rugby player.

Repeated subclinical trauma to any joint can lead to premature cartilage loss with the development of classical osteoarthritis as is shown in the radiograph of the right hip of a 35-year-old squash player (Figure 8.11). This man had been playing the game to a high standard for well over 20 years and was still very active in the sport but complained of persistent pain after matches.

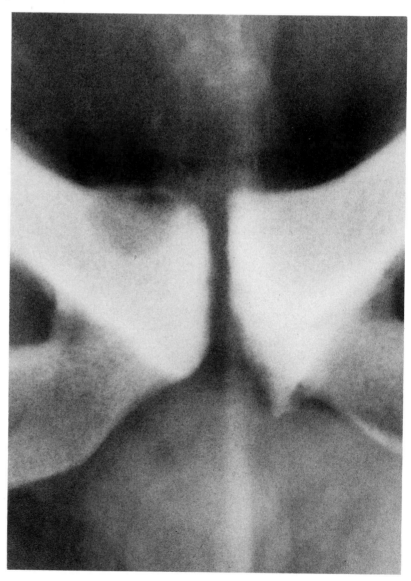

Figure 8.4. Localized view of the symphysis pubis showing sclerosis and cyst formation together with erosions and osteophytes due to chronic osteitis pubis.

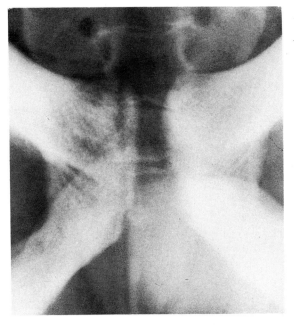

Standing on left leg   Standing on right leg

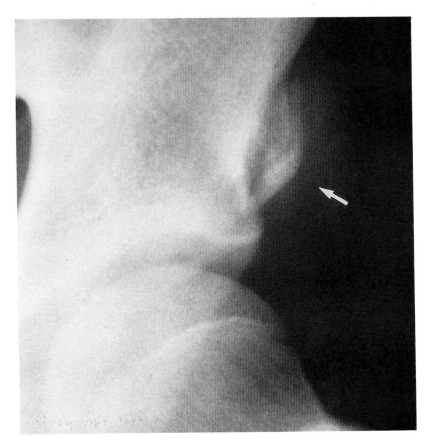

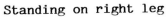

Figure 8.5. (Above). 'Flamingo' views of the symphysis pubis showing mild instability.

Figure 8.6. (Left). Localized view of the left hip in a 14-year-old. There is avulsion of the anterior inferior iliac spine.

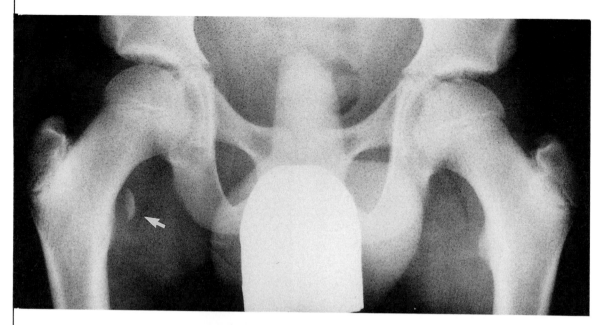

Figure 8.7. (Above). Anteroposterior view of the pelvis in a young male. There is avulsion of the lesser trochanter of the right femur.

Figure 8.8. (Right). Coned view of the same patient illustrated in Figure 8.7, demonstrating the avulsion of the lesser trochanter.

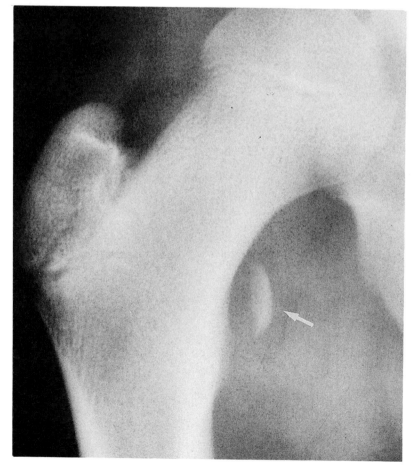

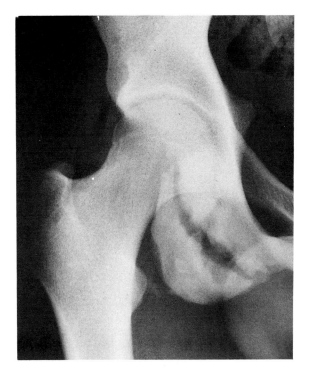

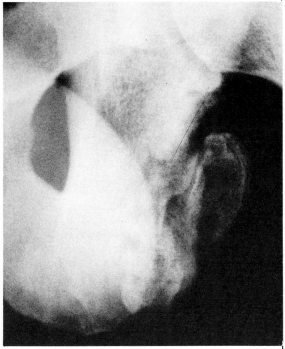

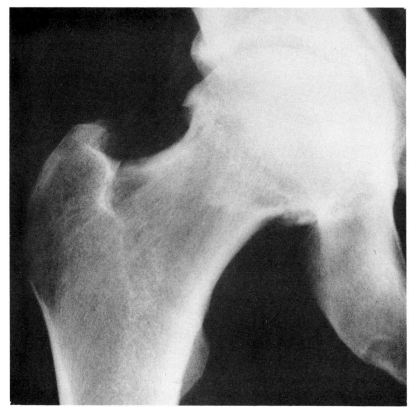

Figure 8.9. (Above left). Anteroposterior view of the right hip of a young adult male. This is a long-standing avulsion of the ischial tuberosity.

Figure 8.10. (Above right). Coned view of the left ischial tuberosity in a young man. There are multiple detached bone fragments with well corticated margins, indicating that this is a long-standing avulsion problem.

Figure 8.11. (Left). Anteroposterior view of the right hip of a 35-year-old man, demonstrating quite marked osteoarthritis with cartilage loss and osteophyte formation.

• BIBLIOGRAPHY •

Adams, R. J. and Chandler, F. A. (1953) Osteitis pubis of traumatic etiology. *J. Bone Joint Surg.* **35(A)**, 658.

Baer, S. and Shakespear, D. (1984) Stress fracture of the femoral neck in a marathon runner. *Br. J. Sports Med.* **18**, 42.

Buckley, S. L. and Burkus, J. K. (1987) Computerized axial tomography of pelvis ring fractures. *J. Trauma* **27**, 496.

Butler, J. E., Brown, S. L. and McConnell, B. G. (1982) Subtrochanteric stress fractures in runners. *Am. J. Sports Med.* **10**, 228.

Cady, G. W., White, E. S. and LaPoint, J. M. (1975) Displaced fatigue fracture of the femoral neck. *J. Bone Joint Surg.* **57(A)**, 1022.

Clancy, W. and Foltz, A. S. (1976) Iliac apophysitis and stress fractures in adolescent runners. *Am. J. Sports Med.* **4**, 214.

Devas, M. B. (1965) Stress fractures of the femoral neck. *J. Bone Joint Surg.* **47(B)**, 728.

Ernst, J. (1964) Stress fractures of the neck of the femur. *J. Trauma* **4**, 71.

Feinbach, S. K. and Wilkinson, R. H. (1981) Avulsion injuries of the pelvis and proximal femur. *Am. J. Radiol.* **137**, 581.

Godshall, R. W. and Hansen, C. A. (1973) Incomplete avulsion of a portion of the iliac epiphysis. An injury of young athletes. *J. Bone Joint Surg* **55(A)**, 1301.

Hanson, P. G. (1978) Osteitis pubis in sports activities. *Phys. Sports Med.* **6**, 111.

Harris, N. H. (1974) Lesions of the symphysis in athletes. *Br. Med. J.* **4**, 211.

Ilsrud, M. E. (1986) Osteitis pubis. *J. Am. Podiat. Med. Ass.* **76**, 562.

Ishikawa, K., Kai, K. and Mizuta, H. (1988) Avulsion of the hamstring muscles from the ischial tuberosity. *Clin. Orthop.* **232**, 153.

Kaltsas, D-S. (1981) Stress fractures of the femoral neck in young adults: a report of seven cases. *J. Bone Joint Surg.* **63(B)**, 33.

Klinefelter, E. W. (1950) Osteitis pubis. Review of the literature and report of a case. *Am. J. Roentgenol.* **63**, 368.

Koch, R. A. and Jackson, D. W. (1981) Pubic symphysitis in runners. A report of two cases. *Am. J. Sports Med.* **9**, 62.

Latshaw, R. F., Kantner, T. R., Kalenak, A., Baum, S. and Corcoran, J. J. Jr. (1981) A pelvic stress fracture in a female jogger: a case report. *Am. J. Sports Med.* **9(1)**, 54.

Lombardo, S. J. and Benson, D. W. (1982) Stress fractures of the femur in runners. *Am. J. Sports Med.* **10**, 219.

Martin, P. (1988) Basic principles of nuclear medicine techniques for detection and evaluation of trauma and sports medicine injuries. *Semin. Nucl. Med.* **18(2)**, 90.

Martin, T. A. and Pipkin, G. (1957) Treatment of avulsion of the ischial tuberosity. *Clin. Orthop.* **10**, 108.

Meurman, K. O. A. (1980) Stress fracture of the pubic arch in military recruits. *Br. J. Radiol.* **53**, 521.

Murray, R. O. and Duncan, C. (1971) Athletic activity in adolescence as an aetiological factor in degenerative hip disease. *J. Bone Joint Surg.* **53(B)**, 406.

Ozburn, M. S. and Nichol, J. W. (1981) Pubic ramus and adductor insertion stress fractures in female basic trainees. *Milit. Med.* **146**, 332.

Panush, R. S., Schmidt, C., Caldwell, J. R., et al. (1986) Is running associated with degenerative joint disease? *J. Am. Med. Ass.* **255**, 1152.

Pavlov, H., Nelson, T. L., Warren, R. F., et al. (1982) Stress fractures of the pubic ramus. A report of twelve cases. *J. Bone Joint Surg.* **64(A)**, 1020

Provost, R. A. and Morris, J. M. (1969) Fatigue fracture of the femoral shaft. *J. Bone Joint Surg.* **51(A)**, 1969.

Puranen, J., Ala-Ketola, L., Peltokallio, P. and Saarela, J. (1975) Running and primary osteoarthritis of the hip. *Br. Med. J.* **2**, 424.

Reiderberger, Von J., Luschnitz, E. and Bauchspeiss, B. (1967) The pubic adductor syndrome in footballers. *Zentralbl. Chir.* **92**, 2655.

Rogge, E. A. and Romano, R. L. (1956) Avulsion of the ischial apophysis (In: Proceedings of the Western Orthopaedic Association). *J. Bone Joint Surg.* **38(A)**, 442.

Schlonsky, J. and Olix, M. L. (1972) Functional disability following avulsion fracture of the ischial epiphysis. *J. Bone Joint Surg.* **54(A)**, 641.

Schneider, R., Kay, J. J. and Ghelman, B. (1976) Adductor avulsion injuries near the symphysis pubis. *Radiology* **120**, 567.

Sennerich, T., et al. (1987) Apophyseal injuries of the pelvis and tibia in adolescent athletes. *Z. Kinderchir.* **42**, 184.

Shon, R. S. and Micheli, L. J. (1985) The effect of running on the pathogenesis of osteoarthritis of the hips and knees. *Clin. Orthop.* **198**, 106.

Skinner, H. B. and Cook, S. D. (1982) Fatigue failure stress of the femoral neck. A case report. *Am. J. Sports Med.* **10**, 245.

Soudry, M., *et al.* (1985) Avulsion of the ischial tuberosity. *Harefuah* **108**, 291.

Thorne, D. A., *et al.* (1986) Pelvic stress fractures in female runners. *Clin. Nucl. Med.* **11**, 828.

Tountas, A. A. and Waddell, J. P. (1986) Stress fractures of the femoral neck. *Clin. Orthop.* **210**, 160.

Wiley, J. (1963) Traumatic osteitis pubis: the gracilis syndrome. *Am. J. Sports Med.* **11**, 360.

Winkler, A. R., *et al.* (1987) Break dance hip: chronic avulsion of the anterior superior iliac spine. *Paediat. Radiol.* **17**, 501.

Zwas, S. T., Elkanovitch, R. and Frank, G. (1987) Interpretation and classification of bone scintigraphic findings in stress fractures. *J. Nucl. Med.* **28**, 452.

9 The Knee

Due to the immense stresses and strains placed on the knee in competitive sport it is an area of the body that commonly causes problems. The knee joint therefore makes up a significant proportion of the work in any sports medicine practice.

Most fractures involving the knee joint are not difficult to diagnose on routine radiographs, although we have seen fractures of the tibial plateau missed by the inexperienced observer and confusion arising with the bipartite patella. Occasionally, when a fracture extends into the knee, fat from the bone marrow can enter the joint-space giving rise to confusion by apparently producing fluid levels. Figure 9.1 illustrates such a problem in a 34-year-old racing cyclist with a fractured patella. The appearances were initially thought to be due to gas within the joint but needling revealed a typical aspirate. This is normally bloody and, when allowed to stand, the marrow floats to the top looking rather like oil on water due to the sparkling fatty droplets which are particularly noticeable when looked at tangentially.

Osteochondral fractures, in which the articular cartilage and a thin section of the underlying subchondral bone are sheared off, can easily be overlooked on X-ray. They usually occur in young people whose articular cartilage is thick, and a sizeable piece may become detached. Routine plain films can appear normal or there may be a small sliver of bone visible in some views, particularly where the fragments are floating free (Figure 9.2). In this 21-year-old tennis player the piece lies in the suprapatellar pouch; in Figure 9.3, which is a coned view of the joint in a 23-year-old wrestler, a fragment can be seen in the intercondylar notch.

Where fragments remain partially attached visualization can be extremely difficult (Figure 9.4) as can be seen from this film of a 19-year-old squash player. Careful fluoroscopy using magnification was needed to produce this radiograph and also to demonstrate the fracture in Figure 9.5 which occurred in a 20-year-old soccer player who injured his knee playing on artificial turf. These fractures are admittedly relatively small ones, but because they involve the articular surface they are certainly not to be regarded lightly.

Similarly small flake fractures, such as the one illustrated in Figure 9.6, may involve only tiny fragments of bone, but this injury to the head of the fibula indicated underlying damage to a portion of the lateral collateral ligament and there was associated disruption of the anterior cruciate. This injury occurred in a 20-year-old soccer player. Figure 9.7 shows bony damage to the head of the fibula and to the anterior tibial spine which was a manifestation of significant injuries involving the lateral collateral and anterior cruciate ligaments.

Clinical assessment of ligamentous injuries is difficult in the acute stage, and examination under anaesthetic is recommended followed by arthroscopy. After the injury has settled, stressed X-ray views (Figure 9.8) can be obtained without as much protective spasm as might render the examination inadequate. These views were obtained in a 21-year-old judo black belt who had disrupted his medial collateral ligament in a competition eight months previously.

In acute knee injuries a diagnostic aspiration of the joint may be undertaken, perhaps confirming the presence of a haemarthrosis. This procedure often provides significant pain relief, which can allow a more diagnostic examination, and it may be combined with the instillation

Figure 9.1. Lateral 'shoot through' X-ray of the knee showing a transverse fracture of the patella extending into the joint. The fluid level (arrow) is due to fat within the joint and not to air or gas.

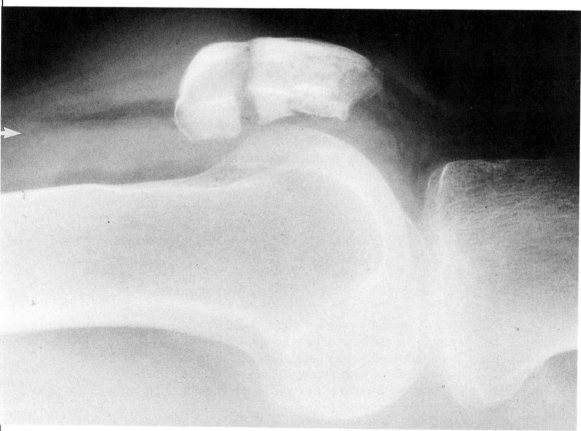

of lignocaine into the joint making for a relatively painless examination of intra-articular structures such as disrupted ligaments.

Figures 9.9(a) and 9.9(b) show normal and stressed views respectively of the knee of a 24-year-old rugby player injured in a tackle which resulted in a disrupted anterior cruciate. As you can see, forward traction of the lower part of the leg with the upper part fixed produced a positive 'drawer' sign. Such a positive drawer sign, done with the knee in flexion, can be elicited only if the hamstrings are not in spasm, and these films were taken with the patient anaesthetized. It is a sign that can be properly demonstrated only when the problem is chronic and therefore not significantly painful. A negative sign does not necessarily mean an intact anterior cruciate but may merely indicate pain and protective spasm.

Where the damage to the ligament is long-standing, as with this 15-year-old rugby player (Figure 9.10), calcification may occur producing the so-called Pellegrini–Stieda lesion, in this case in the distal portion of the medial collateral ligament.

Assessment of the cruciate ligament is possible by arthrography, computed tomography and magnetic resonance imaging. Although these techniques are used extensively in some centres, most orthopaedic surgeons still rely on clinical assessment together, perhaps, with

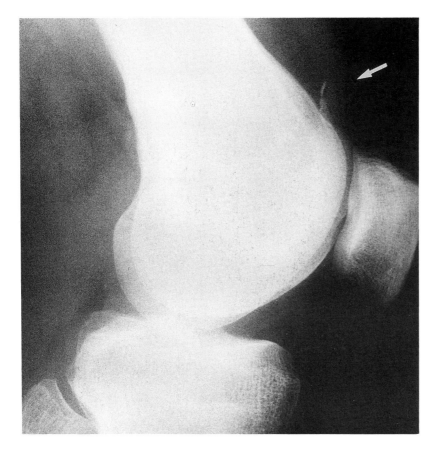

Figure 9.2. Lateral view of the knee showing an osteochondral fragment in the suprapatellar pouch (arrow).

Figure 9.3. Coned view of the intercondylar region of the knee joint showing the tibial spines and a loose osteochondral fragment.

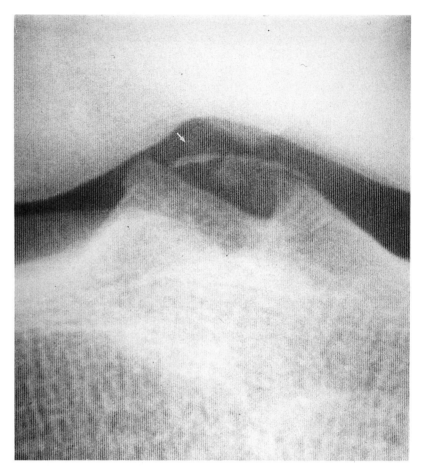

Figure 9.4. Coned view of the medial femoral condyle. The arrow shows a partially detached osteochondral fragment.

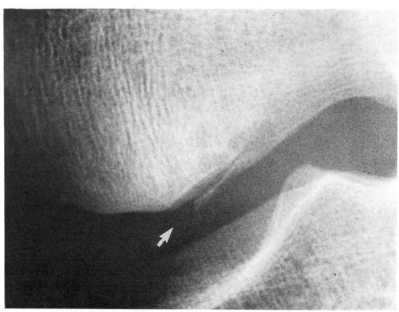

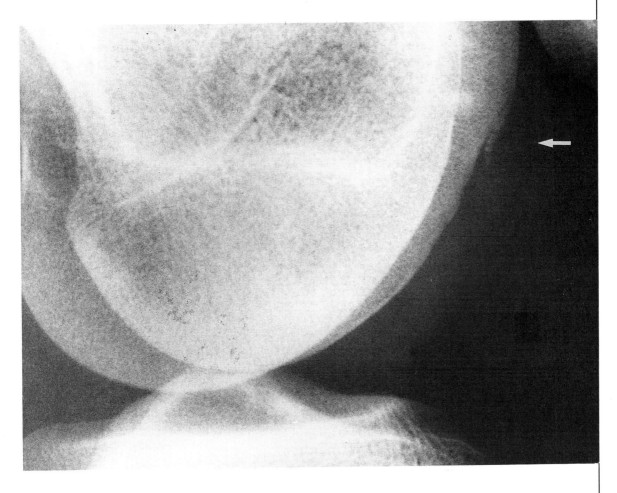

Figure 9.5. Lateral view of the knee. There is a partially detached osteochondral fragment arising from one of the femoral condyles (arrow).

arthroscopy where indicated. Demonstration of the cruciates by arthrography is best done in the lateral position (Figure 9.11). However, it can be very difficult to demonstrate integrity with this technique, while CT scanning of the cruciates is a problem as it is not easy to position the knee within the scanner. MRI scanning may offer a simpler method of investigation as it demonstrates both the anterior and posterior cruciates very well (Figures 9.12 and 9.13), although we feel that clinical assessment of the knee's stability remains important.

Internal derangement of the knee is a common problem in athletes, and the menisci are the structures most commonly involved. Double contrast knee arthrography is a well established and accurate way of assessing the menisci and identifying any damage. The appearances of the normal menisci are shown in Figures 9.14 and 9.15, while Figures 9.16 to 9.21 show a variety of tears. In some centres arthrography is not available and the investigation performed is arthroscopy which in expert hands provides a great deal of information about the internal anatomy of the joint and enables the operator to perform partial menisectomies and other appropriate operative procedures at the same time. It is not difficult, however, for the arthroscopist to miss lesions that can be readily demonstrated on arthrography. In our experience the commonest problem missed is a peripheral detachment of the posterior horn of the medial meniscus (Figures 9.19 and 9.20). We feel that the investigations of arthrography and arthroscopy are complementary and, when used together, result in a very precise diagnosis.

The lateral meniscus is more difficult for the radiologist to demonstrate due to the rather complicated anatomy of the posterior horn and to the relationship of the popliteus tendon, but tears in this region can be revealed by the experienced arthrographer (Figure 9.21).

A congenital anomaly in the knee that can lead to problems is the discoid meniscus, a meniscus that has formed a complete disc instead of having its normal 'C' shape. When this condition presents in adulthood it can be difficult to demonstrate as the meniscus is often thin centrally so that careful examination is needed to show the

Figure 9.6. Small avulsed fragment (arrow) off the head of the fibula indicating damage to part of the lateral collateral ligament.

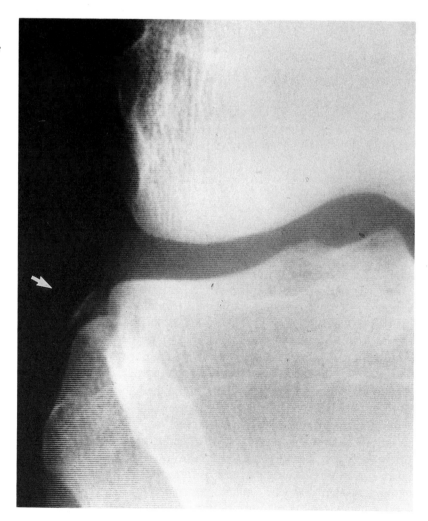

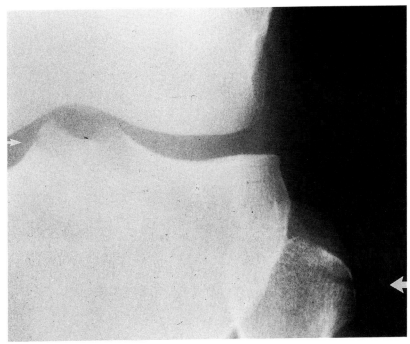

Figure 9.7. Horizontal fracture of the head of the fibula and a fracture of the medial tibial spine in a knee where there was severe disruption of the lateral collateral and anterior cruciate ligaments.

abnormality (Figure 9.22). It is a condition that should always be suspected when young children present with a story suggestive of a torn meniscus, particularly in those under the age of ten years in whom tears to normal menisci are extremely rare. In these children the discoid menisci are fairly obvious, being much larger than normal (Figures 9.23 and 9.24).

With the increasing availability of MRI scanning (Figure 9.25) views of the menisci are becoming more frequently available and attempts to diagnose meniscal tears by this method are underway in several centres.

Recurrent stress injuries to the knee also occur and are usually not too difficult to diagnose. Where the story is suggestive of such a problem and yet routine X-rays are normal, an isotope bone scan may demonstrate abnormal activity related to the excessive stress as shown in Figure 9.26, the positive bone scan of a 34-year-old female marathon runner.

Osteochondritis of the knee is frequently encountered in young teenagers and is probably related to repeated minor trauma; it can be an intractable problem in some cases. The adolescent who presents with anterior knee pain sited below the patella is almost certainly suffering from Osgood–Schlatter's disease, a diagnosis that can usually be made on clinical examination from the soft tissue swelling around, and tenderness of, the tibial tuberosity. It should be noted that the clinical features precede the radiological changes and that comparison views of both knees should be done as the appearances of the tibial tuberosity are variable at this stage. Figures 9.27 and 9.28 show the classical appearances in the normal and affected knees of a 14-year-old long-

Figure 9.8. Stressed view of the knee showing marked widening of the medial compartment due to disruption of the medial ligament. Note that the examiner is unwisely not using protective lead gloves.

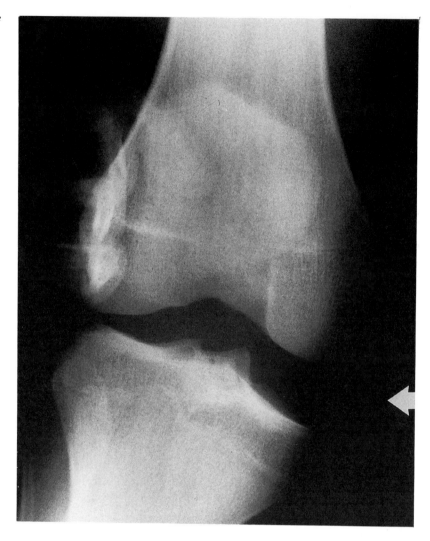

jumper, with soft tissue swelling and marked fragmentation of the epiphysis of the tibial tuberosity. Eventually the condition heals, although it may leave a permanent irregular bony swelling (Figure 9.29) as it has done in the right knee of this 28-year-old hurdler. Occasionally this swelling may be the source of intermittent discomfort at a later age.

In the young teenager who presents with pain and intermittent 'locking' of the knee, an area of osteochondritis dissecans should be suspected. The classical site is the medial femoral condyle as in this young soccer player where a loose fragment of bone has been demonstrated (Figures 9.30 and 9.31). Intercondylar views may be necessary as the abnormal area sometimes lies on this region of the medial condyle (Figure 9.32) and, while this is the condyle most frequently affected, osteochondritis can also be seen on the lateral side (Figure 9.33) as in this tennis player and also occasionally on the posterior surface of the patella (Figure 9.34) as in this young gymnast. The condition may be asymptomatic and is occasionally found purely by chance in a young patient, for instance on plain films to exclude bony damage following an acute knee injury.

Occasionally tomography or CT scanning is used to demonstrate the abnormality, and when MRI facilities are available the lesions can be elegantly shown as they are in Figures 9.35 and 9.36. It is important, however, to remember that irregularity of the femoral condyle in young children is an extremely common finding and osteochondritis should not be readily diagnosed under the age of ten years. When there is any doubt about the diagnosis the safest course is to adopt a 'wait and see' policy as irregular ossification will gradually resolve and osteochondritis dissecans often heals spontaneously in the younger patient. Indeed, the more youthful the athlete the more likely it is that healing will occur. Isotope bone scanning of the condition has been performed but in our experience there is great difficulty in interpreting the films due to the high activity produced by the normal growth plates and the reactive bone about the lesion, although this does not necessarily signify healing.

Arthrography can also be uninformative as the articular cartilage overlying the abnormality may be intact, and this type of lesion may heal with time and decreased stress. Where there is a crack in the hyaline cartilage, this may be demonstrated on MRI or by arthrography; such a lesion will probably not heal because of synovial fluid intrusion. The lesion may become a 'trap-door' type of flap which causes intermittent locking by flipping into the joint, or it may become entirely detached and float around in the cavity as a loose body.

Figure 9.37 shows skyline views of the patellae of a gymnast. While the left is normal, the right shows abnormal calcification in the medial

Figure 9.9. Lateral views of the knee showing a positive 'drawer' sign. (a) The unstressed knee with a normal alignment of the tibia on the femur. (b) Forward displacement of the tibia indicating disruption of the anterior cruciate ligament.

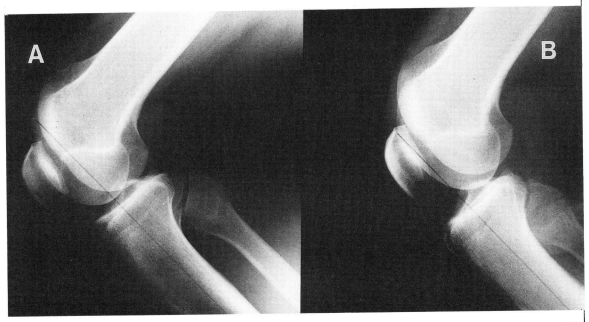

retinaculum which has been torn, and the lateral margin of the lateral femoral condyle demonstrates an osteochondral fracture. These appearances are secondary to an acute dislocation of the patella.

One of the most frequently encountered knee problems in adolescence is chondromalacia patellae, a condition that is commoner in females and that may be due to abnormal tracking of the patella in the intercondylar groove. The diagnosis can usually be made on clinical grounds; routine X-rays are normally of little value, although occasionally minor irregularities or a small area of sclerosis are seen on the posterior surface of the patella (Figure 9.38). Some centres diagnose the condition on arthrography, particularly where this is combined with CT, although our experience at present is that arthroscopy is the investigation of choice where there is doubt on clinical examination.

With the increased demands placed upon top athletes, knee injuries are occurring with worrying frequency. These injuries can lead to chronic instability, resulting in damage to the menisci and articular cartilage and predisposing to the early development of osteoarthritis. Figure 9.39 shows the knee of a 24-year-old rugby player who had an unstable joint following damage to both the medial collateral and anterior cruciate ligaments, and who had undergone a medial meniscectomy. Figures 9.40

Figure 9.10. Faint calcification on the medial side of the tibia (arrow) due to an old injury of the medial ligament (Pellegrini-Stieda lesion).

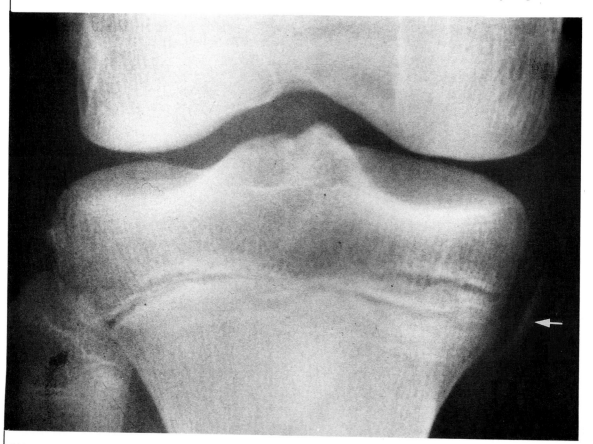

and 9.41 are anteroposterior and lateral views of the knee of a 32-year-old rugby player whose other knee was in only slightly better condition. He had sustained numerous injuries but was still actively playing when these films were taken and reckoned his knees had two or three seasons left in them yet. In patients whose injuries have been of a complex nature involving ligaments and menisci, the degenerative change is often very severe and can present at a relatively early age. It is therefore of great importance that injuries to the knee are fully investigated promptly so that appropriate treatment may be instituted. Fortunately, injuries such as that illustrated in Figure 9.42 are rare. This was sustained by a 30-year-old hang-glider pilot who misjudged a landing, and it ended his sporting career.

The finding of a normal variant on an X-ray is quite common and in asymptomatic patients is unimportant. However, problems occasionally arise where a patient has pain related to this 'normal variant'. The presence of a bi- or tripartite patella (Figures 9.43 and 9.44) is not unusual, and these views were obtained in a 20-year-old field hockey player who complained of pain in the joint after exercise. A bone scan undertaken subsequently (Figure 9.45) showed a marked increase in uptake in the abnormal patella, presumably related to its configuration and aberrant tracking.

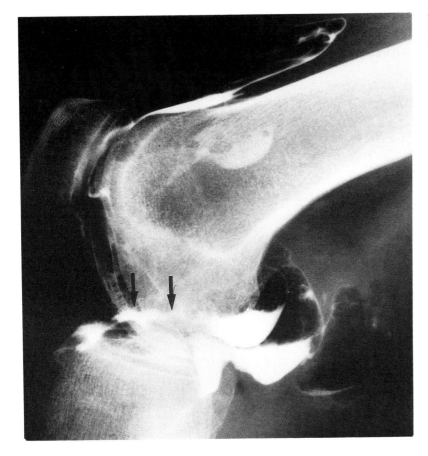

Figure 9.11. Arthrogram of the knee. Lateral view showing the anterior cruciate (arrows).

Figure 9.12. MRI scan of the knee demonstrating a normal anterior cruciate.

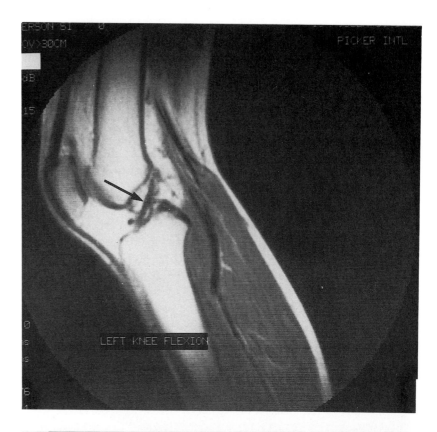

Figure 9.13. MRI scan of the knee demonstrating a normal posterior cruciate.

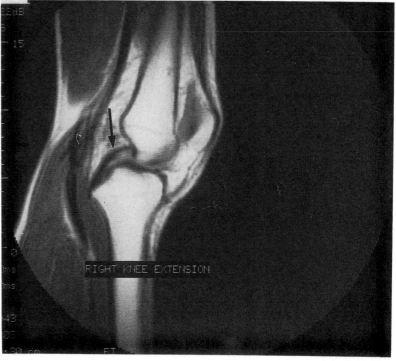

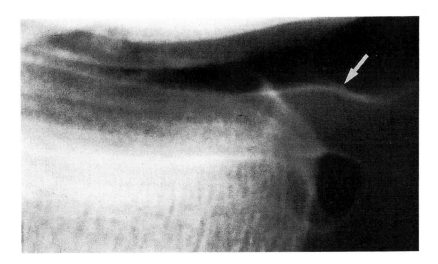

Figure 9.14. Double contrast arthrogram showing a normal anterior horn of the medial meniscus (arrow).

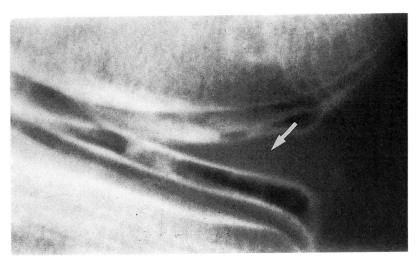

Figure 9.15. Arthrogram demonstrating the normal posterior horn of the medial meniscus (arrow).

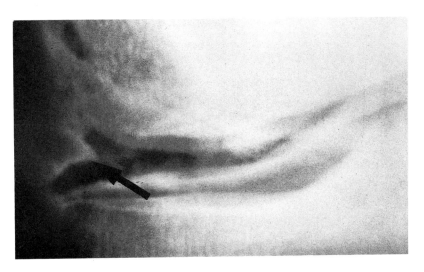

Figure 9.16. Arthrogram showing a severely torn medial meniscus with a small peripheral remnant (arrow).

Figure 9.17. Arthrogram. There is a large tear of the medial meniscus with a displaced fragment (arrow).

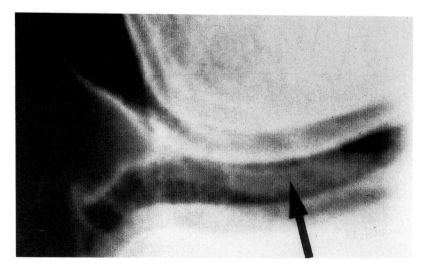

Figure 9.18. Arthrogram showing a horizontal tear of the medial meniscus (arrow). Note the marked widening of the joint space when stressed, indicating laxity of the medial ligament.

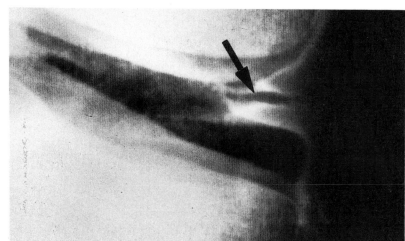

Figure 9.19. Arthrogram showing a peripheral tear of the posterior horn of the medial meniscus. No displacement.

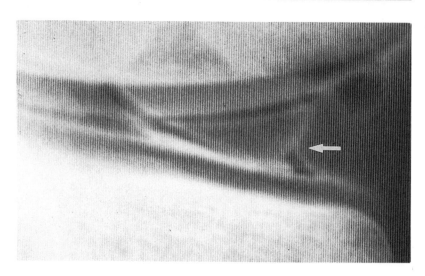

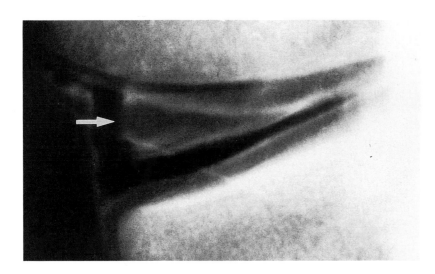

Figure 9.20. Further stress to the knee of the patient in Figure 9.19 has displaced the posterior horn showing a wide gap at the tear (arrow).

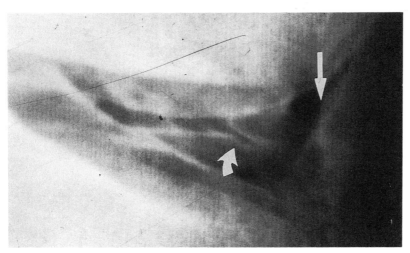

Figure 9.21. Arthrogram showing the posterior horn of the medial meniscus. Note the popliteus bursa (straight arrow) and also a horizontal tear of the meniscus (curved arrow).

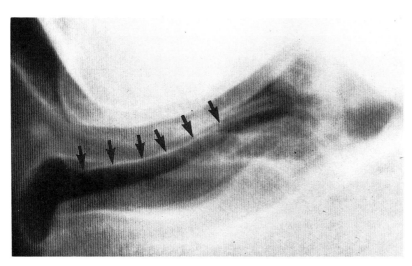

Figure 9.22. Arthrogram of an adult showing a discoid meniscus. Note the continuity of the meniscus from the periphery to the mid-line (arrows).

115

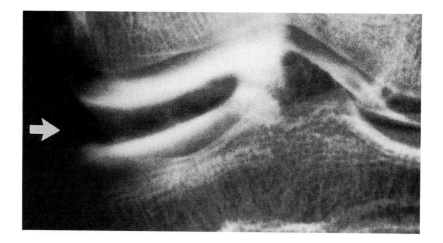

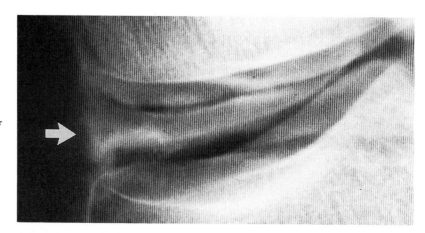

Figure 9.23. (Right). Single contrast arthrogram in a juvenile showing a classical discoid lateral meniscus.

Figure 9.24. (Below right). Discoid lateral meniscus in a double contrast knee arthrogram in a teenager.

Figure 9.25. (Bottom left). MRI scan of the knee demonstrating the posterior horn of a meniscus.

Figure 9.26. (Bottom right). Isotope bone scan of the knee of a female marathon runner. There is markedly increased isotope uptake on the medial tibial condyle due to abnormal stress thought to be in the region of the insertion of the semimembranosus tendon.

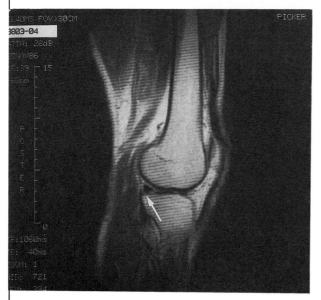

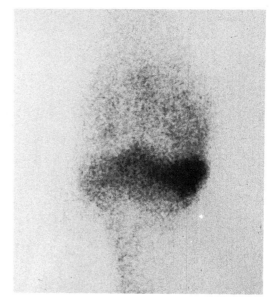

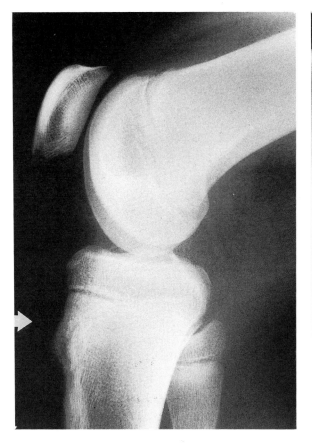

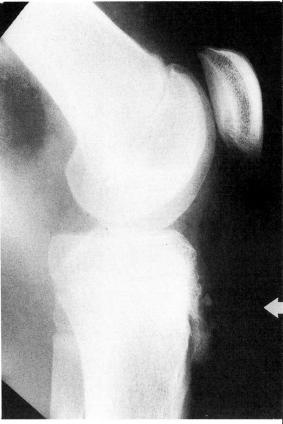

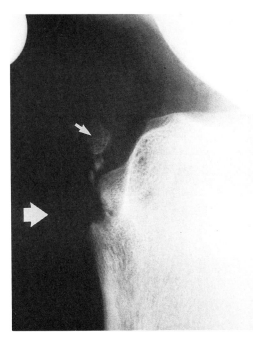

Figure 9.27. (Above left). Lateral X-ray of left knee in a teenager, showing the normal tibial tuberosity.

Figure 9.28. (Above right). Lateral X-ray of the right knee in a teenager (same case as Figure 9.27) showing a fragmented tibial tuberosity due to Osgood–Schlatter's disease.

Figure 9.29. (Left). Deformity of the tibial tuberosity (large arrow) with multiple bone fragments of the patellar insertion (small arrow) due to old Osgood–Schlatter's disease.

117

Figure 9.30. Anteroposterior view of the knee in a 14-year-old boy showing a rather ill-defined area of irregularity on the medial femoral condyle (arrow).

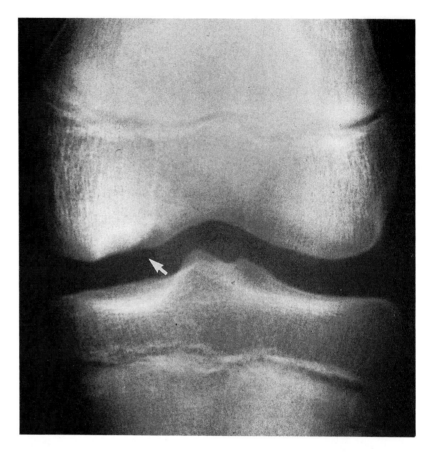

Figure 9.31. Lateral tomogram of the same patient clearly demonstrating a large osteochondral defect due to osteochondritis dissecans (arrow).

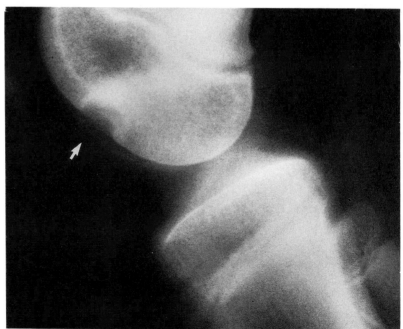

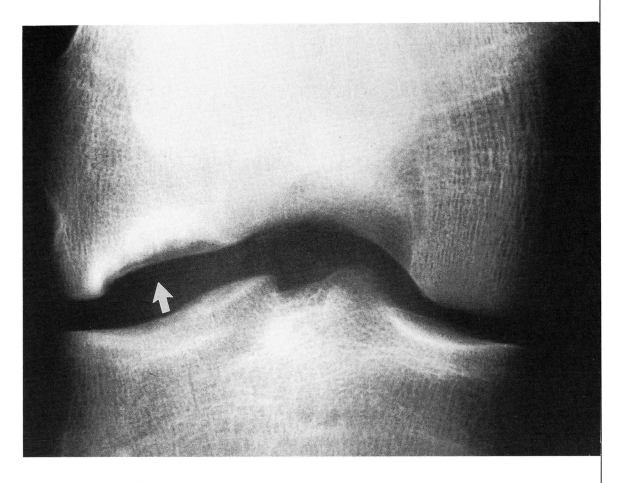

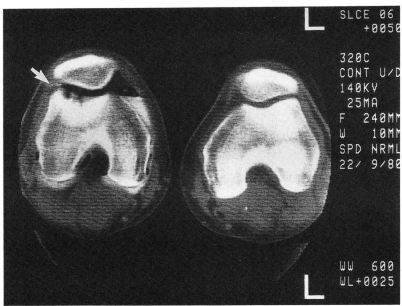

Figure 9.32. (Above). Twenty-year-old squash player with a large established area of osteochondritis dissecans on the medial femoral condyle (arrow).

Figure 9.33. (Left). CT scan of the knees done after a right arthrogram. There is an area of osteochondritis dissecans affecting the lateral femoral condyle (arrow).

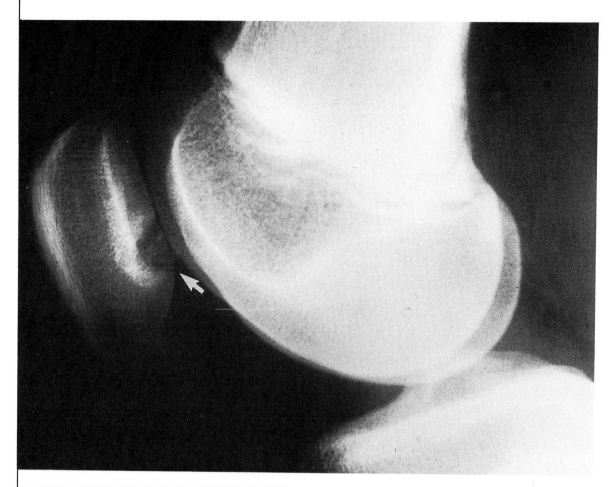

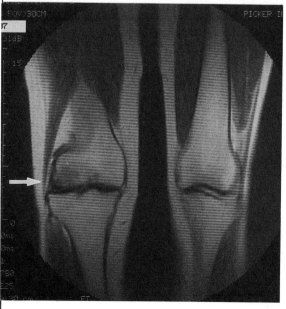

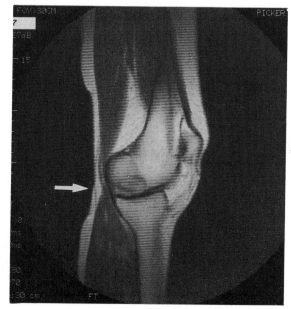

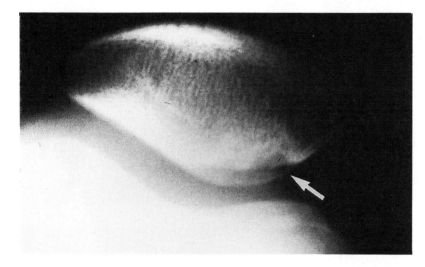

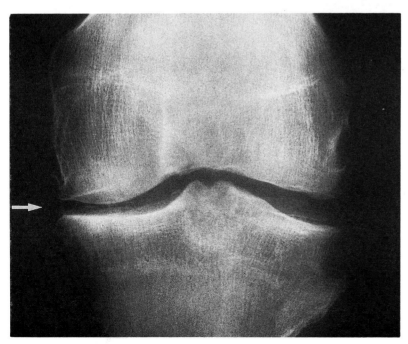

Figure 9.34. (Facing top). Lateral view of the patella showing an area of osteochondritis dissecans (arrow).

Figure 9.35. (Facing bottom left). Anteroposterior view of knees on MRI scan showing a large area of osteochondritis dissecans on the lateral femoral condyle of the knee.

Figure 9.36. (Facing bottom right). MRI scan of the lateral view of the right knee showing an area of osteochondritis dissecans on the lateral femoral condyle (same case as Figure 9.35).

Figure 9.37. (Top). 'Skyline' views of the patellae. The left knee is normal. The right knee shows abnormal ossification in the soft tissues on the medial side of the patella and an area of osteochondritis dissecans on the lateral femoral condyle (arrow).

Figure 9.38. (Above left). 'Skyline' view of the knee showing irregularity of the medial articular surface of the patella due to chondromalacia patellae.

Figure 9.39. (Left). Marked osteoarthritis of the medial compartment in a man aged 24 years. Note the narrowing of the joint space on the medial side (arrow) with osteophytes. This athlete had undergone previous medial meniscectomy.

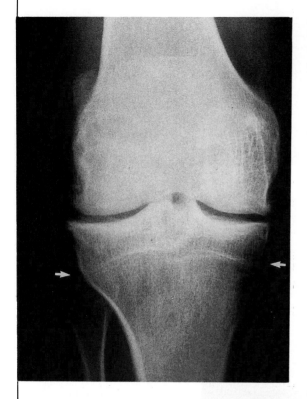

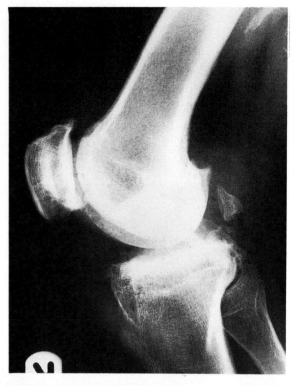

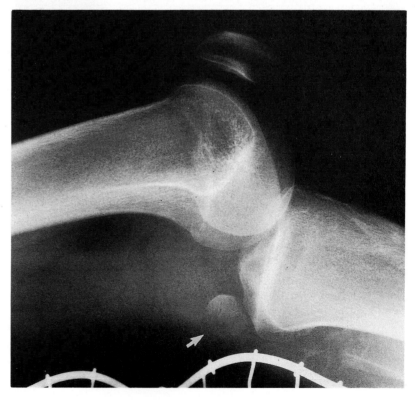

Figure 9.40. (Above left). Anteroposterior view of the knee in a 32-year-old man. Note the epiphyseal lines are still visible (arrows) yet there is marked loss of cartilage in both medial and lateral compartments with osteophytes.

Figure 9.41. (Above right). Lateral view of the same knee showing loose bodies and severe osteoarthritis. This is the end result of many previous sporting injuries.

Figure 9.42. (Right.) Lateral view of the knee showing a disorganized joint with avulsion of the head of the fibula (arrow) and posterior dislocation of the tibia.

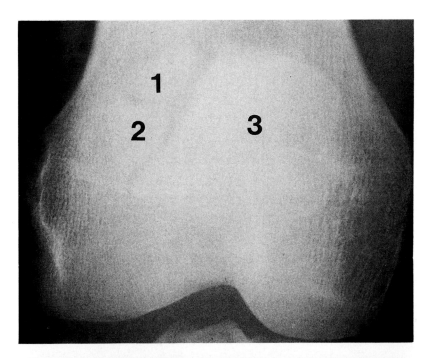

Figure 9.43. (Left). Magnified anteroposterior view of a left knee showing a tripartite patella in the typical site at the upper lateral quadrant of the bone.

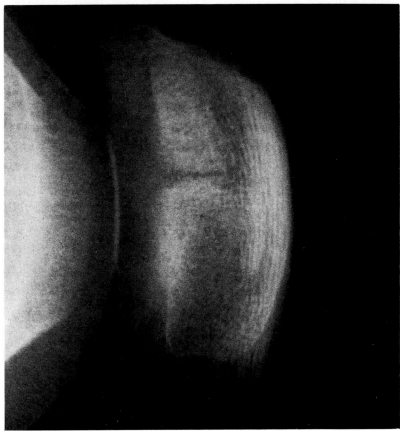

Figure 9.44. (Below). A lateral view of Figure 9.43 showing the abnormality in the bone involving the articular surface.

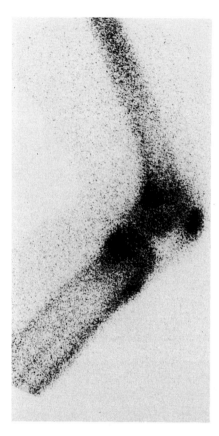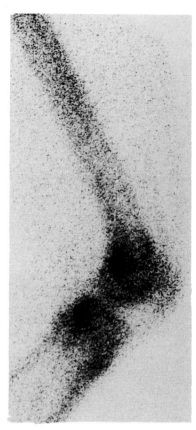

Figure 9.45. Isotope bone scans of the case illustrated in Figure 9.44. The lateral views of the knees are shown; the right side is normal but there is a marked increase of uptake in the left patella.

● BIBLIOGRAPHY ●

Anderson, P. W. and Maslin, P. (1974) Tomography applied to knee arthrography. *Radiology* **110**, 271.

Barrie, H. J. (1987) Osteochondritis dissecans 1977–1987. *J. Bone Joint Surg.* **69(B)**, 693.

Bentley, G. (1970) Chondromalacia patellae. *J. Bone Joint Surg.* **52(A)**, 221.

Berattstrom, H. (1964) Shape of the intercondylar groove normally and in recurrent dislocation of patella: a clinical and X-ray anatomical investigation. *Acta Orthop. Scand.* **68**, 1.

Brown, D. W., Allman, F. L. and Eaton, S. B. (1978) Knee arthrography: a comparison of radiographic and surgical findings in 295 cases. *Am. J. Sports Med.* **6(4)**, 165.

Burry, H. C. (1987) Sport, exercise and arthritis. *Br. J. Rheumat.* **26**, 386.

Butt, W. P. (1987) Soft tissue injuries of the knee—imaging. *Curr. Orthop.* **1**, 145.

Cahill, B. (1985) Treatment of juvenile osteochondritis dissecans and osteochondritis of the knee. *Clin. Sports Med.* **4**, 367.

Carson, W. G., James, S. L., Larson, R. L., *et al.* (1984) Patello-femoral disorders—physical and radiographic examination. Part II—Radiographic examination. *Clin. Orthop.* **185**, 178.

Chick, R. R. and Jackson, D. N. (1978) Tears of the anterior cruciate ligament in young athletes. *J. Bone Joint Surg.* **60(A)**, 970.

Clanton, T. O., DeLee, J. C., Sanders, B. and Neidre, A. (1979) Knee ligament injuries in children. *J. Bone Joint Surg.* **61(A)**, 1195.

Clanton, T. O. and DeLee, J. C. (1982) Osteochondritis dissecans: history, pathophysiology and current treatment concepts. *Clin. Orthop.* **167**, 50.

Dandy, D. J. (1986) *Arthroscopic Management of*

the Knee, 2nd edn. Edinburgh: Churchill Livingstone.

Dalinka, M. K. (1980) Knee arthrography. In: Dalinka, M. K. *Arthrography*. 1st edn. p. 1 New York: Springer.

Darracott, J. and Vernon-Roberts, B. (1971) The bony changes in "chondromalacia patellae". *Rheum. Phys. Med.* **11**, 175.

DeHaven, K. E. (1980) Diagnosis of acute knee injuries with hemarthrosis. *Am. J. Sports Med.* **8**, 9.

DeHaven, K. E., Dolan, W. A. and Mayer, P. J. (1979) Chondromalacia patellae in athletes: clinical presentation and conservative management. *Am. J. Sports Med.* **7**, 5.

Desai, S. S., Patel, M. R., Michelli, L. J., Silver, J. W. and Lidge, R. T. (1987) Osteochondritis dissecans of the patella. *J. Bone Joint Surg.* **69(B)**, 320.

Devas, M. B. (1960) Stress fractures of the patella. *J. Bone Joint Surg.* **42(B)**, 71.

Drez, D. (1985) Arthroscopic evaluation of the injured athlete's knee. *Clin. Sports Med.* **4**, 275.

Edlund, G., Gedda, S. and Hemborg, A. (1980) Knee injuries in skiing: a prospective study from northern Sweden. *Am. J. Sports Med.* **8**, 411.

Ehrenborg, G. (1962) The Osgood–Schlatter lesion. A clinical study of 170 cases. *Acta Chir. Scand.* **124**, 89.

Ellasser, J. C., Reynolds, F. C. and Omohondro, J. R. (1974) The non-operative treatment of collateral ligament injuries of the knee in professional football players. *J. Bone Joint Surg.* **56(A)**, 1185.

Feagin, J. A. Jr. and Curl, W. W. (1976) Isolated tear of the anterior cruciate ligament: 5-year follow-up study. *Am. J. Sports Med.* **4**, 95.

Floyd, A., Phillips, P., Khan, M. R. H., Webb, J. N., McInness, A. and Hughes, S. P. F. (1987) Recurrent dislocation of the patella. *J. Bone Joint Surg.* **69(B)**, 790.

Fulford, P. (1969) Chondromalacia of the patella. *Br. J. Sports Med.* **4**, 198.

Gibson, T., Davies, J. E., Crane, J. and Henry, A. N. (1987) Knee pain in sports people—a prospective study. *Brit. J. Sports Med.* **21**, 115.

Graham, G. P. and Fairclough, J. A. (1988) Early osteoarthritis in young sportsmen with severe anterolateral instability of the knee. *Injury* **19(4)**, 247.

Green, G. P. (1966) Osteochondritis dissecans of the knee. *J. Bone Joint Surg.* **48(B)**, 82.

Guhl, J. (1985) A review of treatment for osteochondritis dissecans. *Contemp. Orthop.* **11(6)**, 19.

Hartzman, S., Reicher, M. A., Bassett, L. W., Duckwiler, G. R., Mandelbaum, A. and Gold, R. H. (1987) M.R. Imaging of the knee. Part II. Chronic Disorders. *Radiology*, **162**, 553.

Havarson, J. B. and Rein, B. I. (1970) Lateral discoid meniscus of the knee. Arthrographic diagnosis. *Am. J. Roentgenol.* **109**, 581.

Heywood, A. W. B. (1961) Recurrent dislocation of the patella: a study of its pathology and treatment in 106 knees. *J. Bone Joint Surg.* **43(B)**, 508.

Holden, D. L. and Eggert, J. E. (1983) The non-operative treatment of Grade I and II medial collateral ligament injuries to the knee. *Am. J. Sports Med.* **11**, 340.

Horns, J. W. (1977) The diagnosis of chondromalacia by double contrast arthrography of the knee. *J. Bone Joint Surg.* **59(A)**, 119.

Hughston, J. C. (1969) Subluxation of the patella in athletes. In: *Symposium on Sports Medicine.* St. Louis: C. V. Mosby.

Insall, J., Falvo, K. A. and Wise, D. W. (1979) Chondromalacia patellae. *J. Bone Joint Surg.* **58(A)**, 1.

Ireland, J., Trickey, E. L. and Stoker, D. J. (1980) Arthroscopy and arthrography of the knee: a critical view. *J. Bone Joint Surg.* **62(B)**, 1.

Jackson, J. P. (1968) Degenerative changes in the knee after meniscectomy. *Br. Med. J.* **2**, 525.

Jacobsen, K. (1977) Osteoarthritis following insufficiency of the cruciate ligaments in man. *Acta Orthop. Scand.* **48**, 520.

Jensen, J. E., *et al.* (1985) Systematic evaluation of acute knee injuries. *Clin. Sports Med.* **4**, 295.

Johnson, L. (1981) *Diagnostic and Surgical Arthroscopy.* St. Louis: C. V. Mosby.

Johnson, R. J., Pope, M. H., Weisman, G., *et al.* (1979) Knee injury in skiing. *Am. J. Sports Med.* **7**, 321.

Keene, G. C. R., Paterson, R. S. and Teague, D. C. (1987) Advances in arthroscopic surgery. *Clin. Orthop.* **224**, 64.

Klunder, K. B., Rud, B. and Hansen, J. (1980) Osteoarthritis of the hip and knee joint in retired football players. *Acta Orthop. Scand.* **51**, 925.

Lane, N. E., Bloch, D. A., Jones, H. H., Marshall, W. H., Wood, P. D. and Frieds, J. F. (1986) Long-distance running, bone density and osteoarthritis. *J. Am. Med. Ass.* **255**, 1147.

Linden, B. (1977) Osteochondritis dissecans of the femoral condyles. *J. Bone Joint Surg.* **59(A)**, 769.

Lipscomb, P. R. Jr., Lipscomb, P. R. and Bryan,

125

Bryan, R. S. (1978) Osteochondritis dissecans of the knee with loose fragments *J. Bone Joint Surg.* **60(A)**, 235.

Lutter, L. D. (1985) The knee and running. *Clin. Sports Med.* **4**, 685.

McPhee, I. B. and Fraser, J. C. (1981) Stress radiography in acute ligamentous injuries of the knee. *Injury* **12**, 383.

Manco, L. G., Kavanaugh, J. H., Lozman, J., Colman, N. D., Bilfield, B. S. and Fay, J. J. (1987) Diagnosis of meniscal tears using high-resolution computed tomography. *J. Bone Joint Surg.* **69(A)**, 498.

Medlar, R. C., Mandiber, J. J. and Lyne, E. D. (1980) Menisectomies in children. Report of long-term results (mean 8.3 years) of 26 children. *Am. J. Sports Med.* **8(2)**, 87.

Micheli, L. J. and Smith, A. D. (1982) Sports injuries in children. *Curr. Probl. Paediatr.* **12**, 2.

Mink, J. H. and Dickerson, R. (1980) Air or CO_2 for knee arthrography. *Am. J. Roentgenol.* **134**, 991.

Noyes, F. R., Mooar, P. A., Matthews, D. S., *et al.* (1983) The symptomatic anterior cruciate deficient knee: the long-term functional disability in athletically active individuals. *J. Bone Joint Surg.* **65(A)**, 154.

Orava, S. and Vitanen, K. (1982) Osteochondroses in athletes. *Br. J. Sports Med.* **16**, 161.

Osgood, R. B. (1903) Lesions of the tibial tubercle occurring during adolescence. *Boston Med. J.* **148**, 114.

Owre, A. (1936) Chondromalacia patellae. *Acta. Clin. Scand.* **77**, 41.

Panush, R. S., Schmidt, C., Caldwell, J. R., *et al.* (1986) Is running associated with degenerative joint disease? *J. Am. Med. Ass.* **255**, 1152.

Passariello, R., Trecco, F., de Paulis, F., Masciocchi, C., Bonanni, G. and Zobel, B. B. (1985) Meniscal lesions of the knee joint: CT diagnosis. *Radiology* **157**, 29.

Pavlov, H. (1983) The radiographic diagnosis of the anterior cruciate ligament deficient knee. *Clin. Orthop.* **172**, 57.

Pavlov, H. and Freiberger, R. H. (1978) An easy method to demonstrate the cruciate ligaments by double contrast arthrography. *Radiology* **126**, 817.

Pavlov, H., Hirschy, J. C. and Torg, J. S. (1979) Computed tomography of the cruciate ligaments. *Radiology* **132**, 389.

Rand, J. A. (1984) The role of arthroscopy in the management of knee injuries in the athlete. *Mayo Clin. Pract.* **59**, 77.

Reicher, M. A., *et al.* (1986) Meniscal injuries: detection using M.R. Imaging. *Radiology* **159**, 753.

Reicher, M. A., *et al.* (1987) M.R. Imaging of the knee. Part I. Traumatic disorders. *Radiology* **162**, 547.

Reider, B., Marshall, J. L. and Warren, R. F. (1980) Clinical characteristics of patellar disorders in young athletes. *Am. J. Sports Med.* **9**, 270.

Reynolds, F. C. (1969) Diagnosis of ligamentous injuries of the knee. In: *Symposium on Sports Medicine.* St. Louis: C. V. Mosby.

Rickards, D. and Chapman, J. A. (1984) Computed tomography of the anterior cruciate ligament. *Clin. Radiol.* **35**, 327.

Robinson, A. R. and Darracot, J. (1970) Chrondromalacia patellae. *Ann. Phys. Med.* **10**, 286.

Seidenstein, H. (1957) Osteochondritis dissecans of the knee: spontaneous healing in children. *Bull. Hosp. Joint Dis.* **18**, 123.

Sisto, D. J. and Warren, R. F. (1985) Complete knee dislocation. *Clin. Orthop.* **198**, 94.

Smillie, I. S. (1957) Treatment of osteochondritis dissecans. *J. Bone Joint Surg.* **39(B)**, 248.

Smillie, I. S. (1969) Knee injuries in athletes. *Proc. R. Soc. Med.* **62**, 937.

Smillie, I. S. (1978) *Injuries of the Knee Joint*, 5th edn. Edinburgh: Churchill Livingstone.

Smillie, I. S. (1980) *Diseases of the Knee Joint*, 2nd edn. Edinburgh: Churchill Livingstone.

Sperryn, P. N. (1983) *Knee Injuries. Sport and Medicine*, 2nd edn, p. 189. London: Butterworths.

Steiner, M. E. and Granan, W. A. (1988) The young athlete's knee: Recent advances. *Clin. Sports Med.* **7(3)**, 527.

Stoker, D. J., Enton, B. and Fulton, A. (1981) The value of arthrography in the management of internal derangement of the knee. *Clin. Radiol.* **32**, 557.

Thinj, C. J. P. (1985) Accuracy of double contrast arthrography and arthroscopy of the knee joint. *Skel. Radiol.* **8**, 187.

Tucker, W. E. (1969) Pellegrini–Stieda or post-traumatic para-articular ossification of the medial collateral ligament of the knee. *Br. J. Sports Med.* **4**, 212.

Turner, D. A., *et al.* (1985) Acute injury of the ligaments of the knee: magnetic resonance evaluation. *Radiology* **154**, 717.

Veth, R. P. H. (1985) Clinical significance of knee joint changes after menisectomy. *Clin. Orthop.* **198**, 56.

10 The Tibia and Fibula

Fractures of the two bones of the lower leg occur in many athletic activities, for instance contact sports such as rugby, gridiron football, soccer, and commonly in the winter sports such as skiing. Usually an injury that breaks the tibia also causes the fibula to fracture, although in the so-called 'boot top' fracture of the tibia in skiers it is not uncommon for the fibula to remain intact. Figure 10.1 shows a spiral 'boot top' fracture of the shaft of the tibia with the fibula unbroken. This injury occurred in a 25-year-old skier practising on a dry ski-slope before his holiday. Figure 10.2 illustrates an 'in boot' greenstick fracture in a 13-year-old skier, again without involvement of the fibula, and Figure 10.3 shows another 'boot top' type fracture in a 19-year-old skier with the fibula again characteristically remaining intact.

Occasionally more severe comminuted fractures can be produced as is shown in Figure 10.4. This unpleasant injury was sustained by a 30-year-old downhill skier who ran into trees, and the radiograph demonstrates a large butterfly fragment anteriorly and an associated fracture of the neck of the fibula.

Direct blows to the lower limbs are extremely common in contact sports and usually result in no more than soft tissue bruising which settles quickly. However, those sustained on the lateral side of the lower part of the leg occasionally result in fractures to the fibula. Blows to the exposed medial surface of the tibia only rarely fracture the bone, although occasionally large subperiosteal haematomas result. In the early stages these are not visible on plain X-rays, although bone scans (Figure 10.5) will show a large, diffuse area of increased isotope uptake. Subsequently the haematoma calcifies and later ossifies as shown in Figure 10.6 and it can then be easily demonstrated. This particular injury occurred in a 26-year-old field hockey player who was accidently struck with a hockey stick with considerable force.

Stress fractures to the tibia are common, and as they are healing produce a periosteal reaction such as the one demonstrated in Figure 10.7 which is a xeroradiograph of a leg of a 27-year-old 10 000 metre runner. Xeroradiography may be a useful technique for demonstrating stress fractures as it produces better pictures of the trabecular pattern of the bone; however, it is an expensive investigation.

Where stress fractures occur in children diagnosis can be more difficult, as such lesions present with pain and the X-ray may show an area of abnormal bone texture together with some periosteal reaction (Figures 10.8 and 10.9). These two illustrations are views of a stress fracture to the upper part of the shaft of the tibia in a 14-year-old cross-country runner. Stress fractures of the tibia account for about 20 per cent of such lesions compared with the 25 per cent that occur in the fibula. A careful history must always be taken, seeking evidence of excessive athletic activity which would tend to confirm the appearances as being those of a stress fracture; confusion may arise in the interpretation of

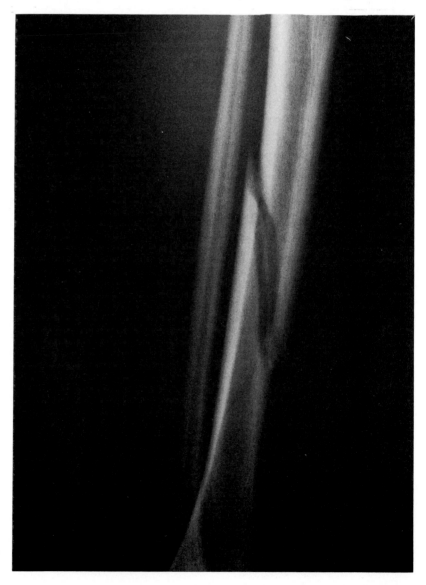

Figure 10.1. Typical spiral fracture of the middle third of the tibia at 'boot top' level. The fibula may remain intact or be fractured at its proximal end.

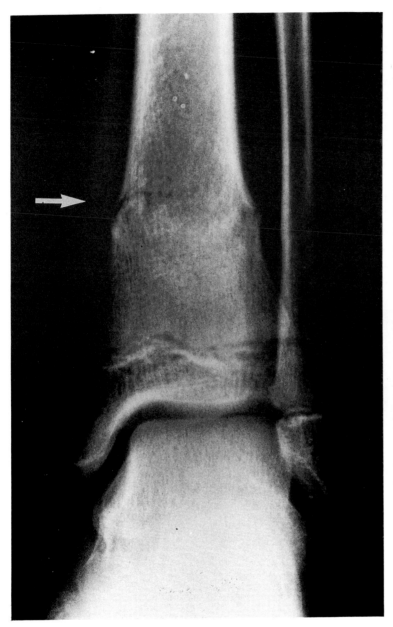

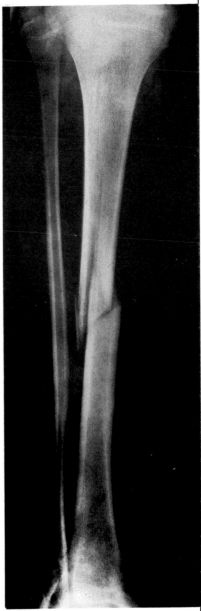

the films since the sites at which stress fractures occur often correspond to those where osteosarcomas may develop. Interpretation of the histology of the tissue obtained at biopsy can be difficult as rapidly proliferating cells will be present in a healing stress fracture. Occasional tragic mistakes have been made.

The radiological clue is that in stress fractures the abnormal sclerosis extends in a linear fashion across the bone. Other investigations at this stage are unrewarding as bone scanning would be abnormal, but where the history is a clear one and the initial radiology is typical, the patient

Figure 10.2. (Above left). Greenstick 'in boot' fracture of the distal third of the tibia in a young skier.

Figure 10.3. (Above right). Typical high 'boot top' fracture of the tibia in a young skier with the characteristically intact fibula.

129

may be reviewed in a few weeks when follow-up X-rays will confirm the presence of a benign stress lesion. Given the drastic consequences of a missed/erroneous diagnosis in this type of case, only the highest standards of history-taking and investigation are acceptable together with careful follow-up.

Fibular stress fractures are again transverse, as is the one shown in Figure 10.10 which occurred in a 28-year-old woman who felt a sharp pain on the outer side of her ankle at the nine-mile stage of a marathon and was forced to pull up shortly thereafter.

An incomplete transverse fracture of the tibia is illustrated in Figure 10.11 and this was sustained by a 21-year-old netball player who, in fact, finished two further matches after the fracture was confirmed. This kind of recklessness can only be most strongly deprecated as disastrous results can follow such behaviour, with complete fracture and delayed union.

When athletes present early with typical pain on exercise and are anxious not to disrupt their training schedules unnecessarily,

Figure 10.4. (Below left). Comminuted fracture of the proximal third of the tibia with a large butterfly fragment and an associated fracture of the neck of the fibula in a downhill skier.

Figure 10.5. (Below right). Isotope bone scan (lateral view) of the lower leg showing diffuse increased activity in the lower third of the tibia due to a subperiosteal haematoma.

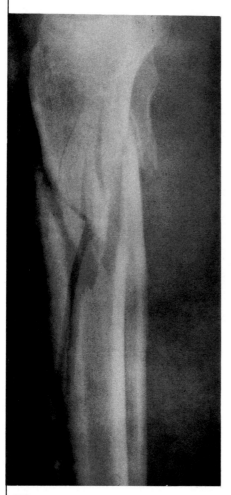

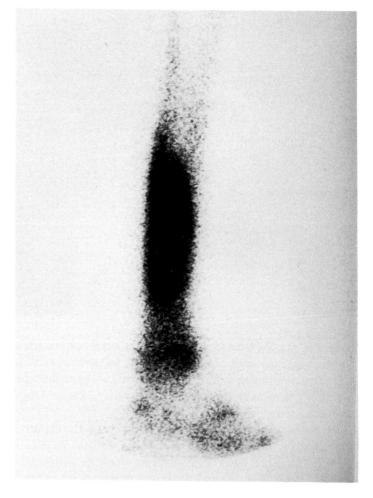

conventional X-rays are rarely helpful: they are almost invariably normal, and a periosteal reaction is not usually visible for some three to four weeks. The diagnostic test of choice in this situation is an isotope bone scan which will demonstrate a stress fracture with high sensitivity even at this early stage. Figure 10.12 shows an isotope bone scan which confirmed the diagnosis of a stress fracture in the left tibia of a 25-year-old 1500 metre runner. Figure 10.13 shows a fibular stress fracture in a 16-year-old 110 metre hurdler.

Another useful investigative technique is the thermogram which identifies areas of increased vascularity such as stress fractures. Figures 10.14 to 10.17 illustrate a series of investigations undertaken in a 29-year-old female middle-distance runner who complained of pain in the lower part of her left leg and ankle on foot strike. Figure 10.14 shows her 'normal' plain X-rays, while Figure 10.15 is a thermogram showing localized hyperaemia over the lower third of the left tibia. A bone scan performed the next day (Figure 10.16) shows a focal area of increased uptake consistent with a stress-related lesion, and this is also illustrated

Figure 10.6. (Below left). X-ray of the tibia of a hockey player (same case as in Figure 10.5) showing organized new bone formation due to a subperiosteal haematoma.

Figure 10.7. (Below right). Xeroradiograph of a healing stress fracture of the tibia showing the periosteal reaction.

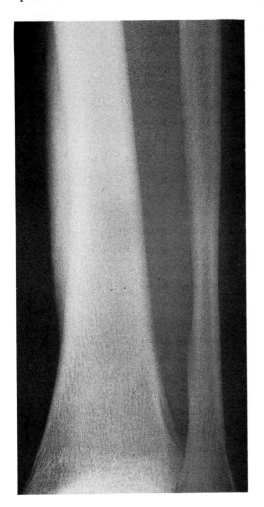

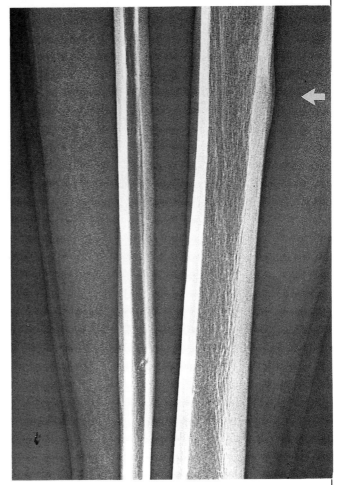

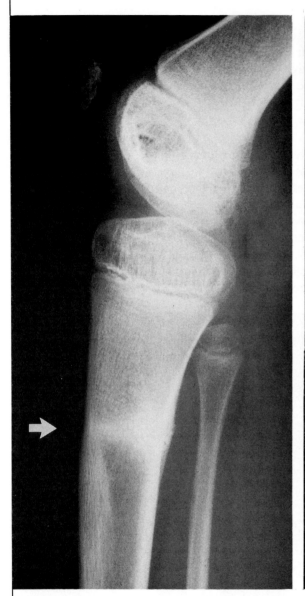

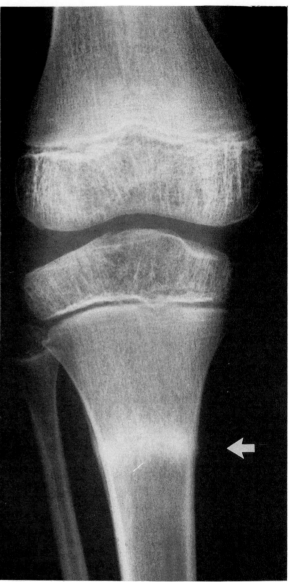

Figure 10.8. (Above left). Lateral view of the knee of a 14-year-old runner showing a stress fracture in the proximal third of the tibia.

Figure 10.9. (Above right). Anteroposterior view of the knee (same case as in Figure 10.8).

in a colourized bone scan (Figure 10.17).

Figure 10.18 shows the plain films of a 35-year-old marathon runner who complained of pain in his right leg after a nine-mile run. The X-rays show a periosteal reaction at the medial border of his right tibia. This man also had a past history of a stress fracture in his left tibia diagnosed some six months before these films were taken. A thermogram (Figure 10.19) showed an area of hyperaemia at the same site as his periosteal reaction and a bone scan (Figure 10.20) demonstrated avid isotope uptake on the right with some residual activity in the left tibia from his previous stress fracture. Figure 10.21 is the colourized version of the bone scan.

Stress fractures show localized areas of abnormal activity, but occasionally diffuse activity over an extended length of bone is also seen. Presumably this is due to abnormal stress throughout the tibia, and such stress may be one of the causes of pain often diagnosed as 'shin splints'. Figure 10.22 is the bone scan of a 24-year-old fast bowler who presented early in the season with lower leg pain, while Figure 10.23 is that of a 20-year-old footballer whose pain came on in pre-season training. In both cases plain films were normal.

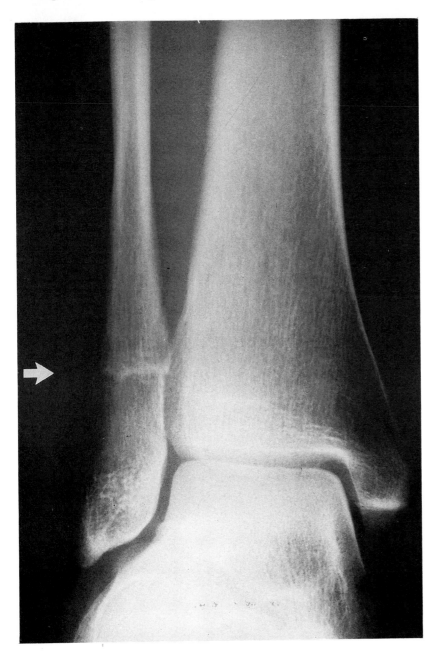

Figure 10.10. Stress fracture of the fibula just above the lateral malleolus in a marathon runner.

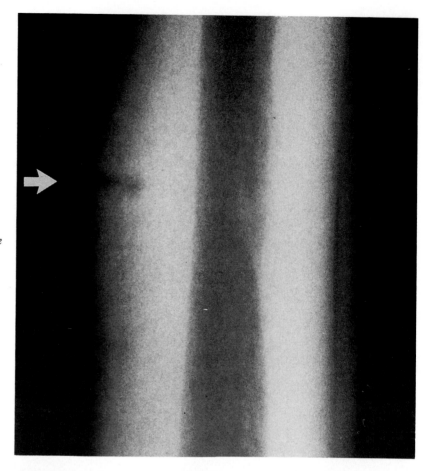

Figure 10.11. (Right). Incomplete stress fracture of the tibia demonstrated using magnification techniques and image intensification.

Figure 10.12. (Below left). Isotope bone scan showing a stress fracture in the left tibia in a 1500 metre runner.

Figure 10.13. (Below right). Bone scan of the lower legs showing a discrete area of abnormal activity in the left fibula at the site of the stress fracture.

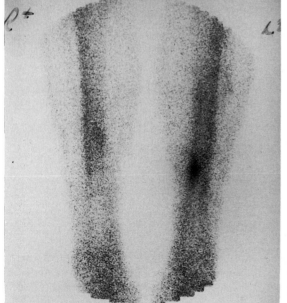

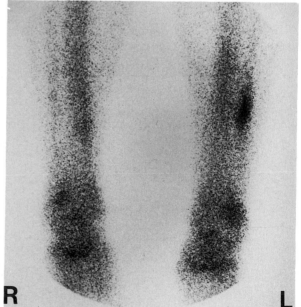

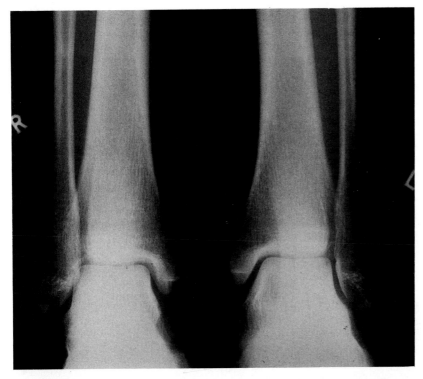

Figure 10.14. (Left). 'Normal' plain X-rays in a 29-year-old international middle-distance runner who complained of pain in the lower third of her left tibia.

Figure 10.16. (Below). Bone scan of athlete (same case as in Figure 10.14) showing a small focal area of increased isotope uptake in the lower third of the left tibia consistent with a stress-related lesion.

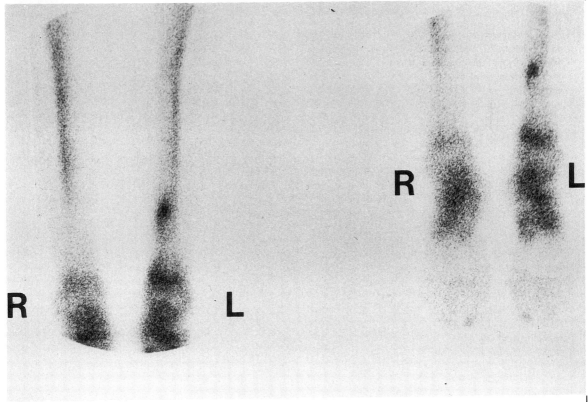

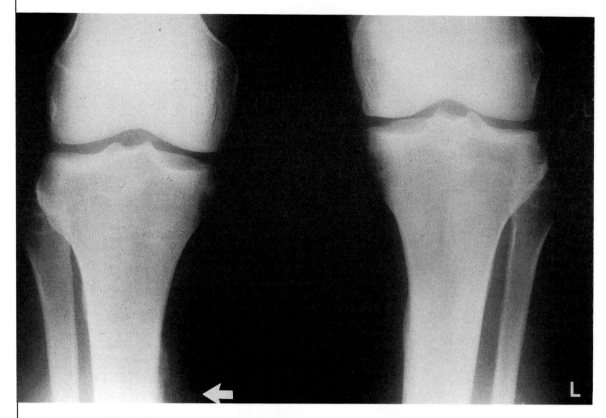

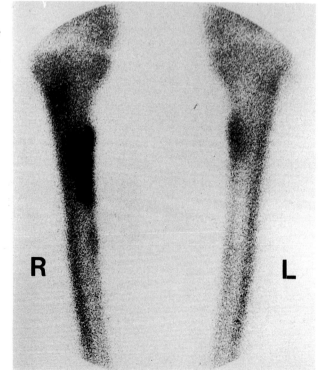

Figure 10.18. (Above). Plain film of knees of a 35-year-old marathon runner showing some periosteal reaction at the medial border of the upper third of the tibia (arrow) due to a stress fracture.

Figure 10.20. (Right). Bone scan of same case as in Figure 10.18 showing avid isotope uptake along the posteromedial aspect of the right upper tibia. There is also a slightly less marked area of excessive uptake in the left tibia at the site of a stress fracture that had occurred six months previously.

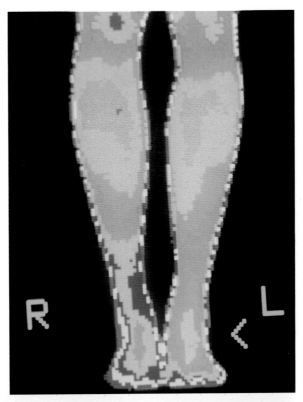

Figure 10.15. Thermogram of athlete (same case as in Figure 10.14) showing localized hyperaemia over anteromedial aspect of lower third of left tibia consistent with periostitis secondary to stress.

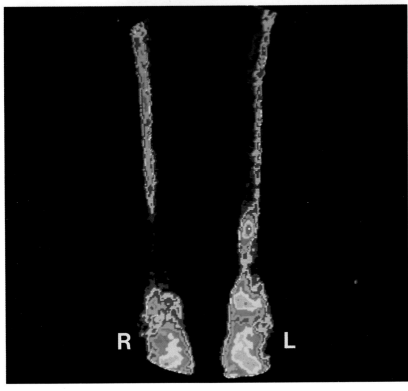

Figure 10.17. Colourized version of the bone scan illustrated in Figure 10.16.

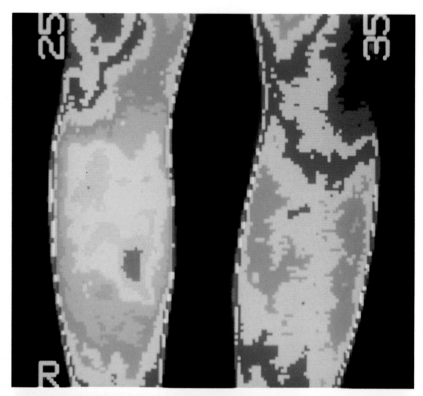

Figure 10.19. Thermogram of same case as illustrated in Figure 10.18 showing an area of hyperaemia over the medial border of the upper tibia.

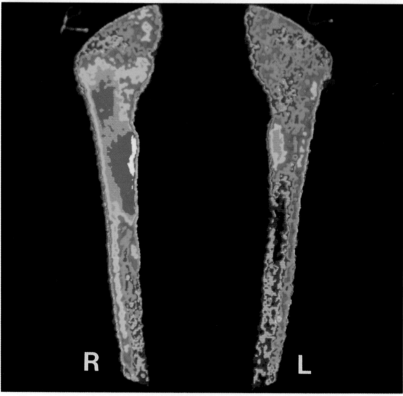

Figure 10.21. Colourized version of the bone scan illustrated in Figure 10.20.

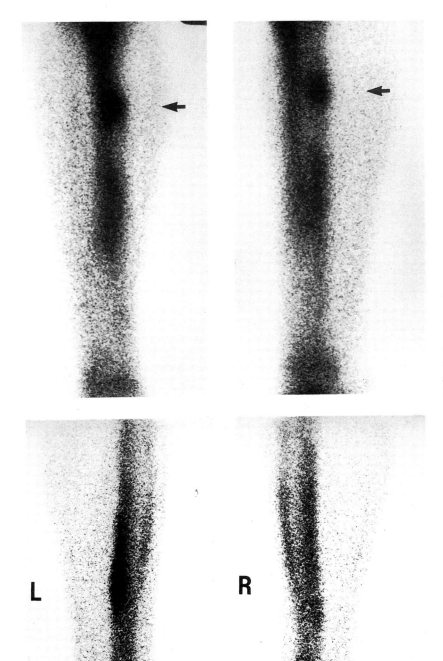

Figure 10.22. Bone scan of the right leg showing diffuse abnormal activity diagnosed as being due to 'shin splints', and also a more discrete area of activity due to a stress fracture. Plain films were normal.

L

R

L R

Figure 10.23. Bone scan of the lower limbs. Lateral projection showing abnormal uptake in both fibulae mainly in the posterior aspect, due to abnormal stress. The left fibula is more affected than the right. Plain films were normal.

137

• BIBLIOGRAPHY •

Belkin, S. A. (1980) Stress fractures in athletes. *Orthop. Clin. N. Am.* **11**, 735.

Brudvig, T. J., Gudger, T. D. and Obermeyer, L. (1983) Stress fractures in 295 trainees: a one-year study of the incidence as related to age, sex, and race. *Milit. Med.* **148**, 666.

Burrows, H. J. (1940) Spontaneous fracture of the apparently normal fibula in its lowest third. *Br. J. Surg.* **28**, 82.

Burrows, H. J. (1950) Fatigue infraction of the middle of the tibia in ballet dancers. *J. Bone Joint Surg.* **38(B)**, 83.

Daffner, R. H., Martinez, S., Gehweiler, J. A. and Harrelson, J. M. (1982) Stress fractures of the proximal tibia in runners. *Radiology* **142**, 62.

Devas, M. B. (1958) Stress fractures of the tibia in athletes or shin "soreness". *J. Bone Joint Surg.* **40(B)**, 227.

Devas, M. B. (1963) Stress fractures in children. *J. Bone Joint Surg.* **45(B)**, 528.

Devas, M. B. (1980) Stress fractures in athletes. *Medisport* **2**, 262.

Devas, M. B. and Sweetman, D. R. (1956) Stress fractures of the fibula. A review of 50 cases in athletes. *J. Bone Joint Surg.* **38(B)**, 818.

Devereaux, M. D., Parr, G. R., Lachmann, S. M., *et al.* (1984) The diagnosis of stress fractures in athletes. *J. Am. Med. Ass.* **252**, 531.

Ellison, A. E. (1977) Skiing injuries. *Clin. Symp.* **29**, 2.

Eriksson, E. and Johnson, R. J. (1981) The etiology of downhill ski injuries. In: Hutton, R. S. and Miller, D. I. (eds) *Exercise and Sport Sciences Reviews.* Philadelphia, Franklin Institute Press 1.

Freeman, J. R., Weaver, J. K., Oden, R. R., *et al.* (1985) Changing patterns in tibial fractures resulting from skiing. *Clin. Orthop.* **216**, 19.

Geslien, G. E., Thrail, J. H., Espinosa, J. L., *et al.* (1979) Early detection of stress fractures using 99mTc-polyphosphate. *Radiology* **121**, 683.

Giladi, M., Milgrom, C., Kashtan, H., Stein, M., Chisin, R. and Dizian, R. (1986) Recurrent stress fractures in military recruits. *J. Bone Joint Surg.* **68(B)**, 439.

Giladi, M., Milgrom, C., Simkin, A., Stein, M., Kashtan, H., Margulies, J., Rand, N., Chisin, R., Steinberg, R., Aharonson, Z., Kedlem, R. and Frankel, V. H. (1987) Stress fractures and tibial bone width. *J. Bone Joint Surg.* **69(B)**, 326.

Gilbert, R. S. and Johnson, H. A. (1966) Stress fractures in military recruits: a review of twelve years' experience. *Milit. Med.* **131**, 716.

Holder, L. E. and Michael, R. H. (1984) Specific scintigraphic pattern of shin splints in lower leg. *J. Nucl. Med.* **25**, 865.

Jaffin, B. (1981) An epidemiologic study of ski injuries: Vail, Colorado. *Mt. Sinai J. Med.* **48(4)**, 353.

Johnson, R. J. and Ettlinger, C. F. (1982) Alpine ski injuries: changes through the years. *Clin. Sports Med.* **1(2)**, 181.

Johnson, R. J. and Pope, M. H. (1977) Tibial shaft fractures in skiing. *Am. J. Sports Med.* **5**, 49.

Johnson, R. J., Ettlinger, M. S., Campbell, R. J. and Pope, M. H. (1980) Trends in skiing injuries: analysis of a 6-year study, 1972–1978. *Am. J. Sports Med.* **8(2)**, 106.

Linscheid, R. L. and Coventry, M. B. (1962) Unrecognized fractures of long bones suggesting primary bone tumours. *Proc. Mayo Clin.* **37**, 599.

Martin, P. (1983) Bone scintigraphy in the diagnosis and management of traumatic surgery. *Semin. Nucl. Med.* **13**, 104.

Maudsley, R. H. (1963) Fatigue fractures of both tibia and fibula. *Postgrad. Med. J.* **36**, 650.

Meurman, K. O. A. and Elfving, S. (1980) Stress fractures in soldiers: multi-focal bone disorders; comparative radiologic and scintigraphic studies. *Radiology* **134**, 483.

Milgrom, C., Giladi, M., Stein, M., *et al.* (1985) Stress fractures in military recruits: a prospective study showing an unusually high incidence. *J. Bone Joint Surg.* **67(B)**, 732.

Nagle, C. E. and Freitas, M. D. (1987) Radionuclide imaging of musculoskeletal injuries in athletes with negative radiographs. *Phys. Sports Med.* **15**, 147.

Ollonquist, L. J. (1929) Callus formation without fracture of shin bones. *Duodecim.* **45**, 473.

Orava, S. (1980) Stress fractures. *Br. J. Sports Med.* **14**, 40.

Renstrom, P. L. and Johnson, R. J. (1985) Overuse injuries in sports: a review. *Sports Med.* **2**, 316.

Rosen, P. R., Micheli, L. J. and Treves, S. (1982) Early scintigraphic diagnosis of bone stress and fractures in athletic adolescents. *Paediatrics* **70**, 11.

Schmitt, M. and Guillot, V. (1984) Thermography and muscular injuries in sports medicine. In: Ring, E. F. J. and Phillips, B.

(eds) *Recent Advances in Medical Thermology*, p. 439–445. New York: Plenum.

Stanitski, C. L., McMaster, J. H. and Scranton, P. E. (1978) On the nature of stress fractures. *Am. J. Sports Med.* **6(6)**, 391.

Sullivan, D., Warren, R. F., Paulou, H., and Kelman, G. (1984) Stress fractures in 51 runners. *Clin. Orthop.* **187**, 188.

Tapper, E. M. (1978) Ski injuries from 1939 to 1976: the Sun Valley experience. *Am. J. Sports Med.* **6**, 114.

Teitz, C. C., Carter, D. R. and Frankel, V. H. (1980) Problems associated with tibial fractures with intact fibulae. *J. Bone Joint Surg.* **62(A)**, 770.

Ungerholm, S., *et al.* (1983) Skiing injuries in children and adults: a comparative study for an eight year period. *Int. J. Sports Med.* **4**, 236.

Van der Linden, W., Sunzel, H. and Larsson, K. (1970) The skiers' boot top fractures. *Acta Orthop. Scand.* **40**, 797.

Washington, E. L. (1978) Musculo-skeletal injuries in theatrical dancers: site, frequency, and severity. *Am. J. Sports Med.* **6**, 75.

Wilcox, J. R., Moniot, A. L. and Green, J. P. (1977) Bone scanning in the evaluation of exercise related stress injuries. *Radiology* **123**, 699.

11   The Ankle

The ankle is the most commonly injured large joint. Most of the injuries affect the soft tissues, are relatively minor, and radiology has little to offer in establishing the diagnosis. However, fractures around the ankle are also extremely common, usually involve the lateral and/or medial malleoli and are easily picked up on normal anteroposterior and lateral radiographs.

Straightforward bimalleolar fractures, such as the one illustrated in Figure 11.1 which occurred in a 26-year-old cross-country runner, are unstable and so are usually, in the UK, internally fixed to prevent them from slipping while they are healing in a cast. As is quite common, the fibular fracture in this man was more easily picked out in the lateral than in the anteroposterior view.

One of the major problems with fractures such as these is an associated ligamentous injury, the most frequent combination being a fracture to the lateral malleolus together with damage to the deltoid ligament medially. Appropriate treatment for these injuries is important at an early stage and careful clinical examination is vital in ensuring a correct diagnosis. The use of arthrography to demonstrate ligament injuries is not a routine procedure in the UK, although it is performed in some centres if it is felt that early diagnosis will affect management, and then it is a useful procedure.

The so-called trimalleolar fracture involving the lateral, medial and posterior malleoli is also always unstable, and is consequently a serious injury. However, isolated fractures of the posterior malleolus (Figure 11.2), although less common, often carry a poor prognosis due to severe damage to the soft tissues and articular cartilage; the dome of the talus and the posterior articular cartilage of the tibia are normally fractured and produce joint irregularities. The one illustrated here was sustained by a 34-year-old basketball player on landing and resulted in his retirement from the game.

Not all ankle fractures stand out, and a cursory glance may miss a small avulsion fracture such as the one illustrated in Figure 11.3 which was causing problems for a 26-year-old fast bowler. The presence of the small fragment shown in fact represented significant damage to the ligament and could not be ignored; inadequate treatment could have led to permanent problems. It can occasionally be difficult to differentiate between accessory ossicles, previous injuries with small detached fragments of bone in the soft tissues, and a new injury. When major clinical doubt exists regarding the diagnosis, a bone scan may be diagnostic (Figure 11.4); increased activity in the area confirms the presence of a recent problem.

The majority of damaged ligaments heal satisfactorily with conservative treatment, but some go on to long-term instability. Because the lateral ligament is the one most frequently damaged, it is at this site that the instability is commonly found, the patient presenting with persistent ankle pain, swelling and recurring injuries. The diagnosis in such cases is confirmed by obtaining positive stress views, ideally done under screening control using image intensification. It is essential that both the normal and the abnormal ankle are examined as some individuals have very lax ligaments.

The owner of the damaged left ankle illustrated in Figure 11.5 was a 24-year-old triple-jumper who had sustained the initial injury some 18 months before these films were taken, and who underwent surgical repair before returning successfully to competitive sport. Unfortunately, it is not unusual for such athletes to sustain similar injuries subsequently,

Figure 11.1. X-ray of unstable bimalleolar fracture in a 26-year-old cross-country runner. The fibular fracture is best seen in the lateral view.

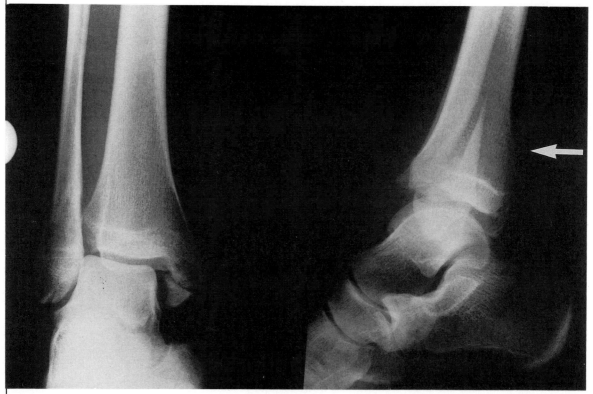

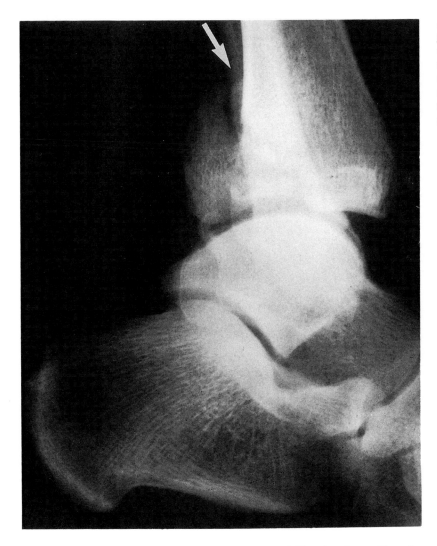

Figure 11.2. Fracture of the posterior margin of the lower end of the tibia (posterior malleolus) with anterior subluxation of the tibia on the talus. Clearly an unstable injury with associated ligament damage.

and Figure 11.6 shows lateral ligament instability in the ankle of a 30-year-old long-jumper who re-injured the joint three years after a satisfactory result from a previous repair. Second repairs are generally more difficult and less successful, and this athlete was unwilling to undergo further surgery at this late stage in his career and subsequently retired.

Our experience is that stress views can be performed in chronic cases without the use of sedation or general anaesthesia although this, or injection of local anaesthetic, has been found to be useful by others if diagnostic films are to be obtained.

Stress problems related to repeated trauma occur commonly, and a striking example is shown in Figure 11.7 in a fast bowler who characteristically dragged his trailing foot before delivering the ball. This has led to a fragment being avulsed off the posterior margin of the talus. The athlete concerned spent his winters playing and coaching

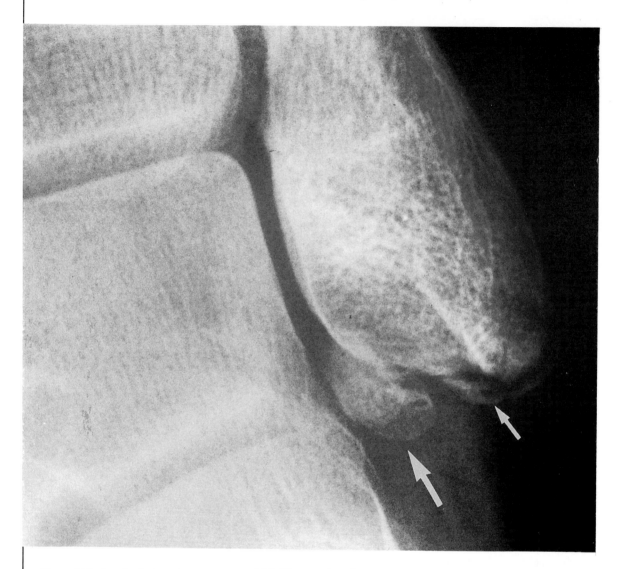

Figure 11.3. Localized view of the lateral malleolus showing an accessory os subfibulare (large arrow) and a small avulsion off the tip of the malleolus (small arrow).

soccer, and his X-rays also show an abnormal bony spur on the anterior superior border of his talus. Although such spurs have been described as normal variants, they have also been noted to be frequently present in footballers, basketball players and gymnasts, even at a very young age. This is the so-called 'footballer's' ankle, and the resultant spurs and tibial osteophytes may well result in an impingement. They are caused by repetitive dorsiflexion injuries and by the collision of the anterior talus and capsule against the anterior border of the distal tibia.

The end-result of repeated minor trauma or a major injury is the development of early osteoarthritis with loss of articular cartilage. Loose bodies may also be present which, if they are radio-opaque, can be shown on plain films (Figure 11.8) or when radiolucent (usually small fragments of cartilage) can be demonstrated by an arthrogram. The ankle in Figure 11.8 is that of a 30-year-old professional footballer who, incidentally, also had quite marked degenerative changes in both knees.

Fractures of the talus are not common (Figure 11.9) but when they occur they are often complicated by severe soft tissue trauma. Even when the fracture is a straightforward one across the neck of the talus, problems may arise with the onset of avascular necrosis at a later date. In the case shown in Figure 11.9 the comminuted fracture to the bone was sustained by a young male gymnast who misjudged a dismount in an unofficial and unsupervised warm-up. Gymnasts place immense strains upon their ankle joints on landing, and disastrous injuries such as this one can easily occur unless the highest safety standards are observed.

Osteochondritis dissecans most commonly affects the knee joint and is illustrated in that chapter; however, it does affect other joints, including the ankle. Osteochondritis is most commonly found in young adult males and involves the superior border of the dome of the talus (Figure 11.10). As in the knee, a fragment may separate and produce an intra-articular loose body with consequent recurrent pain, swelling and locking. The case illustrated was found in a 32-year-old rugby player and, as it is situated on the medial aspect of the joint, may be due to a pronation injury.

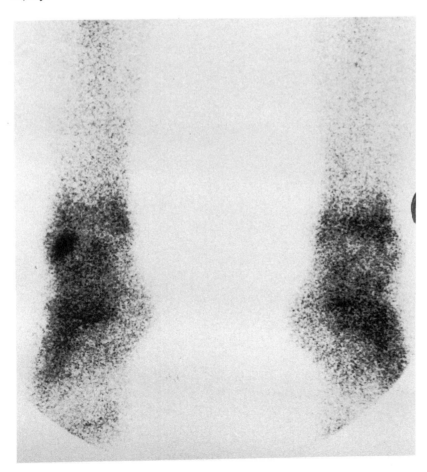

Figure 11.4. Bone scan of the ankles showing increased activity at the tip of the left lateral malleolus. This is a scan of the case shown in Figure 11.3 and confirms the presence of a fracture.

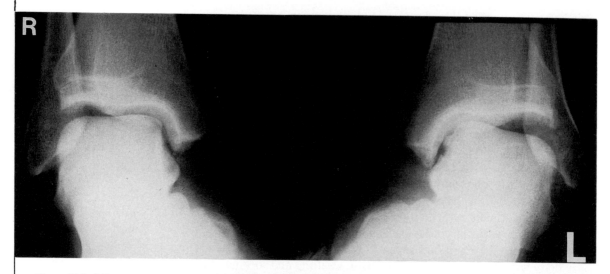

Figure 11.5. (Above). Stress views of the ankles. The right is normal, and the left shows lateral ligament instability.

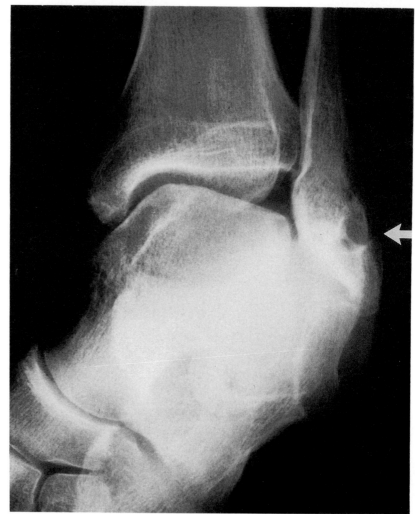

Figure 11.6. (Right). Stress view of the ankle showing lateral ligament instability despite a previous ligament repair. There is a defect in the lateral malleolus at the site of the insertion of the ligament repair (arrow).

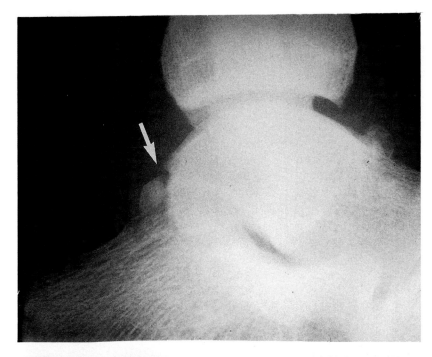

Figure 11.7. Lateral view of the ankle. There is a fragment off the posterior margin of the talus (arrow) and a bony spur on the anterior superior border of the talus causing an impingement.

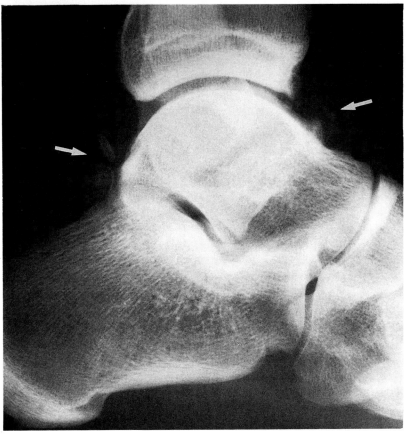

Figure 11.8. Lateral view of the ankle showing signs of chronic damage with bony spurs on the anterior superior surface of the talus and on the anterior border of the distal tibia, with multiple radio-opaque intra-articular loose bodies (arrows).

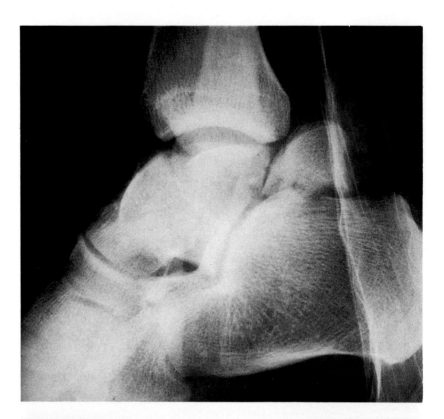

Figure 11.9. Comminuted fracture of the talus.

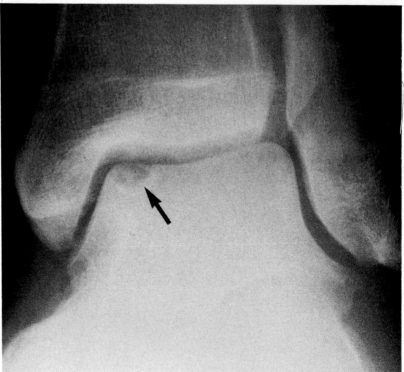

Figure 11.10. View of the ankle showing an area of osteochondritis dissecans on the medial edge of the dome of the talus (arrow).

● BIBLIOGRAPHY ●

Almquist, G. (1974) The pathomechanics and diagnosis of inversion injuries to the lateral ligaments of the ankle. *J. Sports Med.* **2**, 109.

Anderson, K. J., LeCocq, J. F. and Clayton, K. L. (1962) Athletic injury to the fibular collateral ligament of the ankle. *Clin. Orthop.* **23**, 146.

Bauer, M., Jonsson, K. and Linden, B. (1987) Osteochondritis dissecans of the ankle. *J. Bone Joint Surg.* **69(B)**, 93.

Brand, R. L., Black, H. M. and Cox, J. S. (1977) The natural history of inadequately treated ankle sprains. *Am. J. Sports Med.* **6**, 248.

Bromstrom, L. (1965) Sprained ankles. II. Arthrographic diagnosis of recent ligament ruptures. *Acta Chir. Scand.* **129**, 485.

Bromstrom, L. (1966) Sprained ankles. V. Treatment and prognosis in recent ligament ruptures. *Acta Chir. Scand.* **132**, 537.

Canale, S. T. and Kelly, F. B. (1978) Fractures of the neck of the talus. *J. Bone Joint Surg.* **60(A)**, 143.

Comfort, T. H., Behrens, F., Gaither, D. W., Denis, F. and Sigmond, M. (1985) Long term results of displaced talar neck fractures. *Clin. Orthop.* **199**, 81.

Cox, J. S. and Hewes, T. F. (1979) "Normal" talar tilt angle. *Clin. Orthop.* **140**, 37.

Downing, J. W., Oloff, L. M. and Jacobs, A. M. (1979) Radiologic diagnosis and assessment of lateral ankle ligamentous injuries. *J. Foot Surg.* **18**, 135.

Freeman, M. A. R. (1965) Instability of foot after injuries to the lateral ligaments of the ankle. *J. Bone Joint Surg.* **47(B)**, 669.

Flick, A. B. and Gould, N. (1985) Osteochondritis dissecans of the talus (transchondral fractures of the talus): review of the literature and new surgical approach for medial dome lesions. *Foot Ankle* **5**, 165.

Garrick, J. G. and Requa, R. K. (1988) The epidemiology of foot and ankle injuries in sports. *Clin. Sports Med.* **7(1)**, 29.

Gordon, R. B. L. (1970) Arthrography of the ankle joint. Experience in one hundred and seven studies. *J. Bone Joint Surg.* **52(A)**, 1623.

Harrington, K. D. (1979) Degenerative arthritis of the ankle secondary to long-standing lateral ligament instability. *J. Bone Joint Surg.* **61(A)**, 354.

Kaye, J. J. and Bohne, W.H.O. (1977) A radiographic study of the ligamentous anatomy of the ankle. *Radiology* **125**, 659.

Kingston, S. (1988) Magnetic resonance imaging of the ankle and foot. *Clin. Sports Med.* **7(1)**, 15.

Leach, E. and Lower, G. (1985) Ankle injuries in skiing. *Clin. Orthop.* **198**, 127.

Lindstrand, A. (1976) New aspects in the diagnosis of lateral ankle sprains. *Orthop. Clin. N. Am.* **7**, 247.

Mack, R. P. (1975) Ankle injuries in athletics. *Athletic Training* **10**, 94.

McManama, G. B. (1988) Ankle injuries in the young athlete. *Clin. Sports Med.* **7(3)**, 547.

McMurray, T. P. (1950) Footballer's ankle. *J. Bone Joint Surg.* **32(B)**, 68.

Olson, R. W. (1969) Arthrography of the ankle: its use in the evaluation of ankle sprains. *Radiology* **92**, 1439.

Parkes, J. C., Hamilton, W. G., Patterson, A. H. and Arwles, J. G. (1980) The anterior impingement syndrome of the ankle. *J. Trauma* **20**, 895.

Penny, N. and Davis, L. A. (1980) Fractures and fracture-dislocations of the neck of the talus. *J. Trauma* **20**, 1029.

Prins, J. G. (1978) Diagnosis and treatment of injury to the lateral ligament of the ankle. *Acta Chir. Scand.* **486**, 3.

Roden, S., Tillegard, P. and Unander-Scharin, L. (1953) Osteochondritis dissecans and similar lesions of the talus: report of fifty-five cases with special reference to etiology and treatment. *Acta Orth. Scand.* **23**, 51.

Sauser, D. D., Nelson, R. C., Lavine, M. H. and Wu, C. W. (1983) Acute injuries of the lateral ligaments of the ankle: comparison of stress radiography and arthrography. *Radiology* **148**, 653.

Seligson, D., *et al.* (1980) Evaluation of the lateral collateral ligaments. *Am. J. Sports Med.* **8**, 39.

Shelbourne, K. D., *et al.* (1988) Stress fractures of the medial malleolus. *Am. J. Sports Med.* **16(1)**, 60.

Staples, O. S. (1975) Ruptures of the fibular collateral ligaments of the ankle. *J. Bone Joint Surg.* **57(A)**, 101.

12 The Foot

It is the common practice of athletes in many disciplines to run long distances in order to improve their level of fitness and endurance. Consequently foot problems are not just confined to those whose sporting activity involves running.

The biomechanics of the foot are intimately linked with those of the ankle. For anatomical reasons we have split up the two structures, but we are well aware that problems at the ankle can result from an 'abnormal' foot, although deciding exactly what should be called 'abnormal' is often difficult. Certainly great emphasis has been given to the role of excessive pronation in the production of foot problems but there are many factors other than ones of technique and anatomy that produce lesions such as stress fractures. Over-ambitious training schedules, inadequate footwear, and running on inappropriate surfaces such as asphalt rather than grass or Tartan track, can be injurious whilst training, and playing in studded (cleated) footwear on hard, sun-baked or frozen surfaces is also a cause of over-use damage.

Foot problems in dancers occur for similar reasons, i.e. practising on unsuitable surfaces, and over-use injuries are common in that profession.

Foot pain in the athlete has to be properly diagnosed, as stress fractures must be differentiated from soft tissue injuries. Stress fractures are a common problem and certainly need rest, perhaps immobilization, and possibly even internal fixation.

Simple stress fractures of the foot are easily diagnosed by conventional X-rays and most commonly affect the shaft of the second metatarsal. Those that occur at the bases of the metatarsals (Figure 12.1) can be missed due to the overlapping images found on some views of this area. This particular injury occurred in a 10 000 metre runner who trained regularly on roads.

Figure 12.2 illustrates the more common site for stress fractures of the metatarsals (i.e. to the mid-shaft) and this lesion occurred in a cricketer who had been bowling on sun-baked Australian wickets in December and January after a season of county cricket in England. The

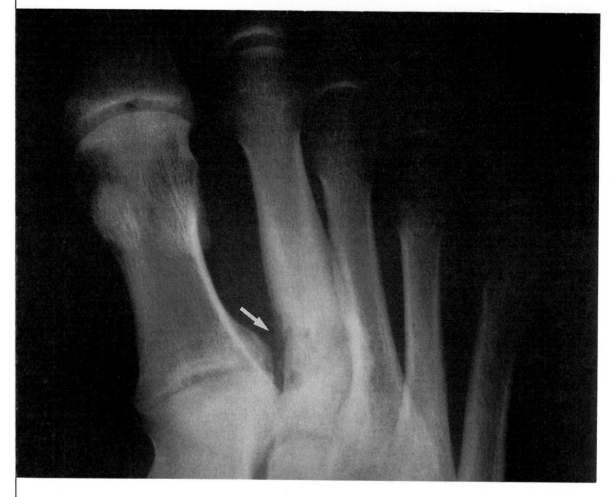

Figure 12.1. X-ray showing a stress fracture of the base of the second metatarsal of the right foot.

fracture was in his left foot as he was a right-arm fast bowler and this foot was, therefore, the one taking the strain in his delivery stride.

Not all stress fractures of the metatarsals are immediately obvious, and Figure 12.3 is a radiograph of the foot of a 240 lb prop forward who, when he returned from playing rugby on hard grounds in Spain for three weeks, complained of foot pain. This film (Figure 12.4) was passed as normal by an inexperienced observer despite the slight periosteal reaction on the shaft of the third metatarsal, which was not commented upon. The isotope bone scan (Figure 12.5) confirms that the abnormality was due to a stress fracture.

The so-called Jones' fracture occurring distal to the tuberosity of the proximal part of the base of the fifth metatarsal is notoriously difficult to treat. Figure 12.6 illustrates such an injury in the foot of a basketball player; these athletes seem to be particularly prone to this lesion. In view of the problems in obtaining adequate healing within a reasonable time in such injuries some orthopaedic surgeons recommend internal fixation of these fractures.

Stress fractures of the tarsal bones most commonly occur in the calcaneum and navicular, and the athlete whose foot is illustrated in Figure 12.7 was an 18-year-old female road runner who presented with foot pain and a history suggestive of a stress fracture. The initial films were normal, but when the foot was manipulated, screened, and the tarsus magnified, the lesion demonstrated in Figure 12.8 was found. Had this not been detected we would have proceeded to isotope bone scanning, which is diagnostic. Figure 12.9 illustrates the positive bone scan of a female marathon runner and demonstrates a stress fracture of the navicular in the right foot. Figure 12.9 also shows that such scans

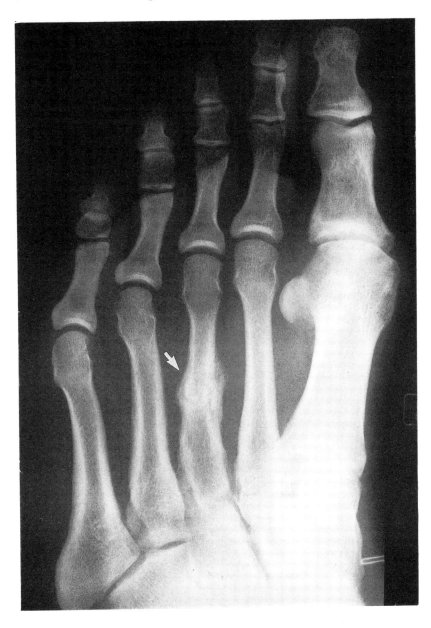

Figure 12.2. X-ray showing a healing stress fracture of the mid-shaft of the third metatarsal of the left foot.

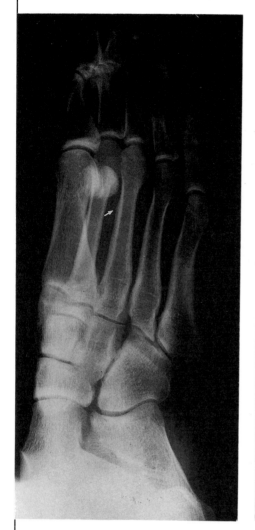

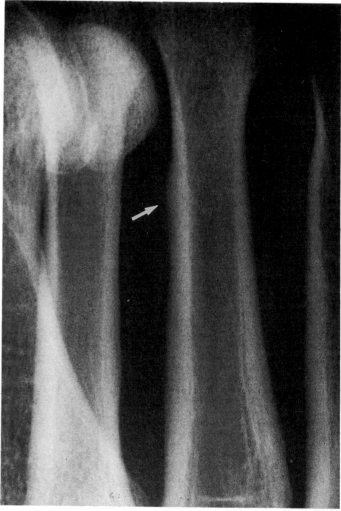

Figure 12.3. (Above left). X-ray of the left foot of a rugby player complaining of foot pain and passed as normal by an inexperienced observer.

Figure 12.4. (Above right). Localized view of the shaft of the third metatarsal showing a slight periosteal reaction (same film as in Figure 12.3).

will readily demonstrate the presence of other 'hot spots' due to the abnormal stresses to which the feet are subjected in these patients.

The consequences of missing a navicular stress fracture can be serious. Figure 12.10 is one of a series of tomograms of the foot of a 25-year-old football player who, being on the fringes of international honours, was playing frequently and training hard. He had sought medical opinion regarding his foot pain, had been reassured, and after a short period of rest continued his sporting activity. Unfortunately, however, the problem worsened to the extent that he had to leave the field at half-time on his international debut. An X-ray taken shortly afterwards was passed as normal and after a further brief period of convalescence he began to play again, attempting to 'play through' the foot pain. As might be expected the pain worsened and he was again forced to seek medical advice when the fracture was demonstrated (Figure 12.10). He subsequently underwent open reduction and screw fixation of the navicular (Figure 12.11), the whole saga having extended over almost two years. The particular tomogram selected shows that the fractured ends of the bone had become widely separated with sclerosis indicating established non-union.

A stress fracture occurring in the cuneiform is illustrated in Figure 12.12 and this was sustained by a 27-year-old boxer who was doing a good deal of road running in inappropriate footwear as part of his pre-fight training. He was subsequently unable to fulfil his commitment as far as this particular bout was concerned since his foot pain impeded his movements around the ring.

Isotope bone scans are extremely useful in the diagnosis of stress injuries; the examination is not an expensive one and the radiation dose is small. However, it should be remembered that although the sensitivity of the test is extremely high its specificity is very low and areas of abnormal uptake may be due to conditions other than stress fractures, such as infection or tumour. It should not therefore be looked upon as an alternative to a good clinical history and thorough physical examination.

The stress fracture of the calcaneum shown in Figure 12.13 was detected after a half-marathon, the 30-year-old runner seeking medical

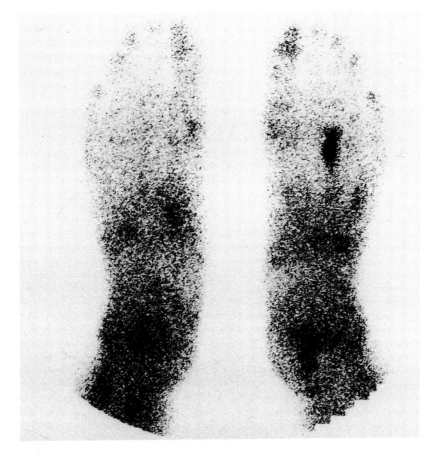

Figure 12.5. Bone scan of feet (same patient as in Figures 12.3 and 12.4) showing a 'hot spot' on the shaft of the left third metatarsal, confirming a stress fracture.

155

advice upon completion of the event. He had experienced pain in the heel while training but was determined to take part and so did not consult a doctor before the start. This is a common story amongst athletes, from those of international standard down to 'fun runners', as all are loathe to interrupt their training schedule without a very good reason.

Heel pain in athletes is a common complaint and is often due to soft tissue injuries such as straightforward bruising. Figure 12.14 shows the lateral view of the right heel of a 41-year-old, rather overweight, jogger who was running 30 miles a week. There is a bony spur and some irregularity of the inferior surface of the calcaneum posterior to this. He was seen complaining of heel pain which came on at about the two-mile mark, and his isotope scan (Figure 12.15) showed grossly abnormal uptake in the calcaneum, the so-called 'jogger's heel'. There was also a hot spot in the distal portion of the fifth metatarsal, an area that was only mildly symptomatic.

Figure 12.16 shows a lateral view of the calcaneum of a 40-year-old ex-international squash player, who still played daily to a high standard and who had a history suggestive of plantar fascitis. The calcaneal spur was noted and a bone scan (Figure 12.17) revealed a hot area around the spur. The patient's symptoms responded satisfactorily to a short period of rest and injection of corticosteroid.

The aetiology of the heel spur is normally calcification due to traction phenomena and necrosis of the plantar fascia as it inserts into the anterior aspect of the calcaneum. Any spur extending in the horizontal plane is normally calcification of the plantar fascia due to necrosis of the tissues from repetitive stress, and one should be very slow to operate on it.

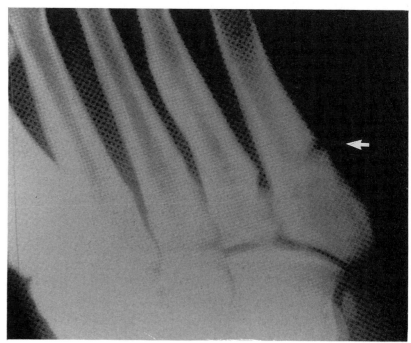

Figure 12.6. Localized view of a stress fracture of the base of the fifth metatarsal (Jones' fracture).

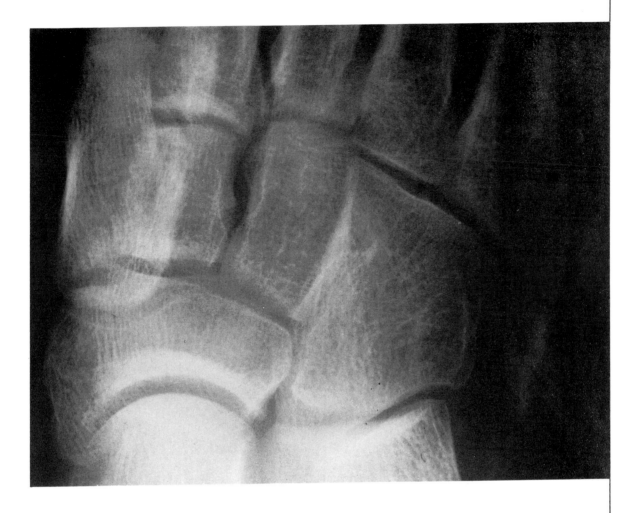

Figure 12.7. Localized view of the tarsus showing an apparently normal navicular.

Those facing plantarward or perpendicular to the longitudinal axis of the calcaneum are often due to direct trauma, perhaps secondary to poor fat-pad coverage. They may well lend themselves to orthoses and occasionally to surgery, but tend to respond poorly to injection.

The osteochondritides (avascular necrosis/aseptic necrosis) are a common but puzzling group of conditions. There is now clear evidence that they are due to an interruption of the blood supply to the bone, and some disorders appear to be related to excessive physical activity.

Figure 12.18 shows a lateral view of the heel and ankle of a 12-year-old netball player who complained of heel pain. She noticed this particularly as it was her main landing foot. Plain X-ray revealed early calcaneal apophysitis (Sever's disease) although these appearances in the absence of symptoms would have been regarded as unremarkable. The treatment of the condition is to reduce stress on the area, stress can be reduced radically by casting, moderately by reducing activity, or functionally by elevating the heel with a heel lift/raise during activity in an effort to change the angle of pull of the tendon on the bone. The

Figure 12.8. X-ray taken using magnification during screening showing a stress fracture completely splitting the navicular (same patient as in Figure 12.7).

Figure 12.9. (Facing top). Isotope bone scan of the feet showing grossly abnormal uptake in the right navicular due to a stress fracture. There are areas of increased activity in both feet, also probably related to abnormal stress.

Figure 12.10. (Facing bottom left). Tomogram of a fractured navicular in the right foot, with wide separation of the fragments and an established non-union.

Figure 12.11. (Facing bottom right). Postoperative reduction and screw fixation of navicular (same patient as in Figure 12.10).

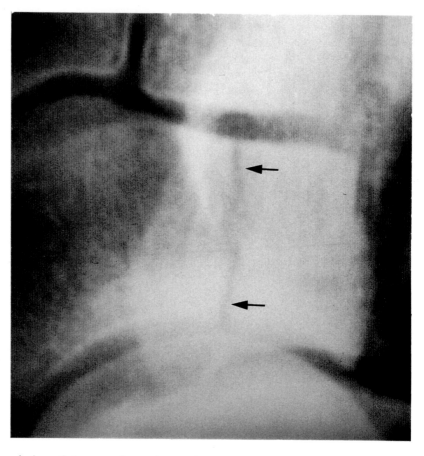

choice of therapy depends on the severity of the symptoms, and the condition generally settles within a few months leaving no permanent sequelae.

Much more dramatic are the appearances of Figure 12.19 which is the foot of a six-year-old ballet dancer who presented with persistent foot pain and whose X-ray revealed osteochondritis of the navicular (Kohler's disease) which was sclerotic and compressed. The disorder nearly always heals without any long-term problems or a residual deformity, although occasionally there may be a slight change in the bony architecture of the foot leading to long-term morbidity.

Finally there is Freiberg's infraction which is illustrated in Figure 12.20. This disorder affects the head of the second metatarsal which collapses and becomes flattened, this occasionally giving rise to osteoarthritis in later life.

Like athletes, dancers frequently impose considerable strains upon their feet. Figure 12.21 illustrates the quite severe osteoarthritic changes found secondary to over-use and repeated minor trauma, in a relatively young (aged 30 years) male dancer. Such problems, which to the athlete can be no more than the source of some discomfort and irritation, can be disastrous to a dancer.

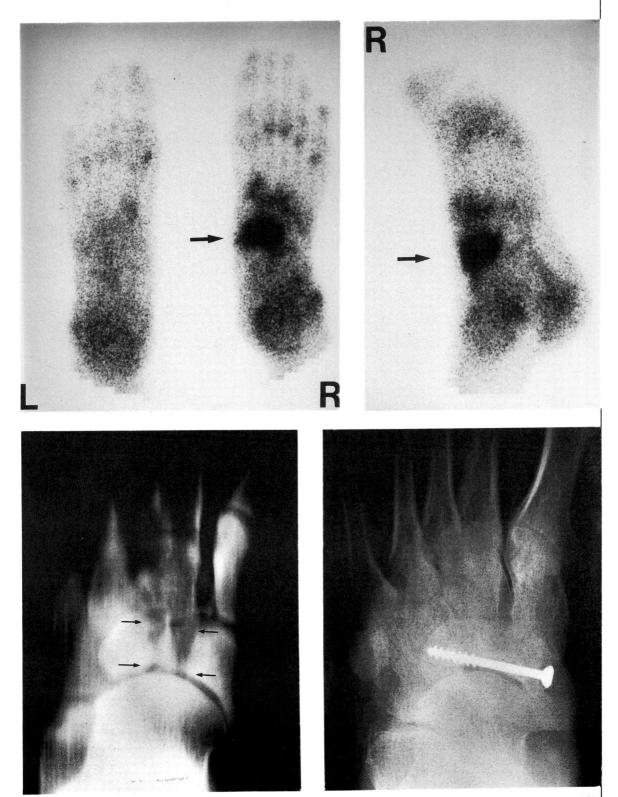

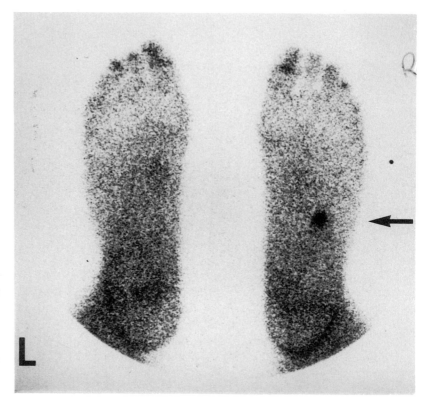

Figure 12.12. (Right). Isotope bone scan of the feet showing an area of abnormal activity in one of the cuneiform bones of the right foot due to a stress fracture. Plain X-rays were normal.

Figure 12.13. (Below). Lateral view of the calcaneum showing a stress fracture in the upper part of the bone posteriorly.

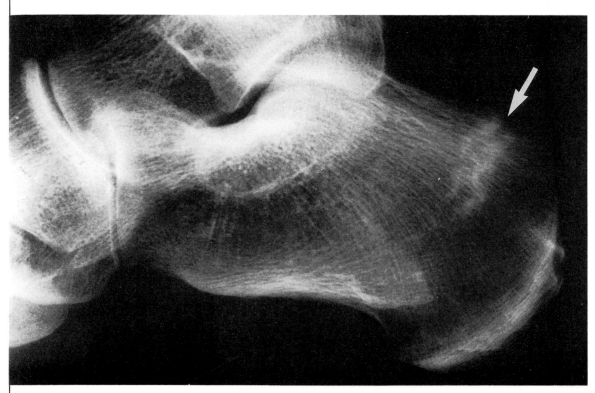

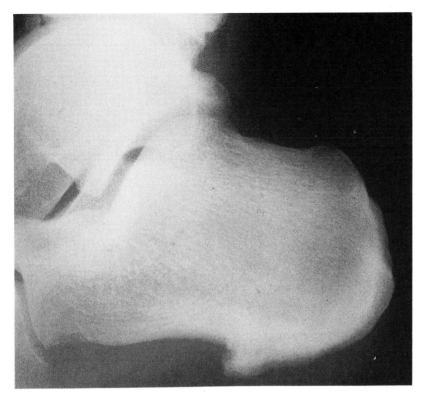

Figure 12.14. (Left). Lateral view of a right heel showing an abnormal bony spur with some irregularity of the inferior surface of the calcaneum posteriorly.

Figure 12.15. (Below). Isotope bone scan of the feet (two views). This is the same case as in Figure 12.14, showing grossly abnormal uptake in the right calcaneum and, incidentally, in the fifth metatarsal.

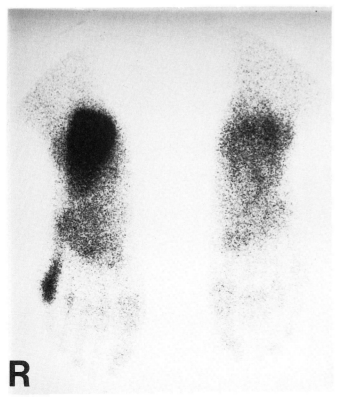

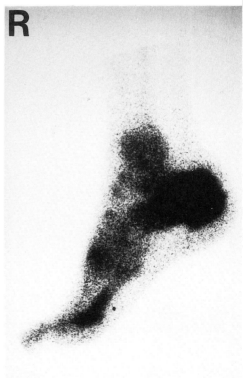

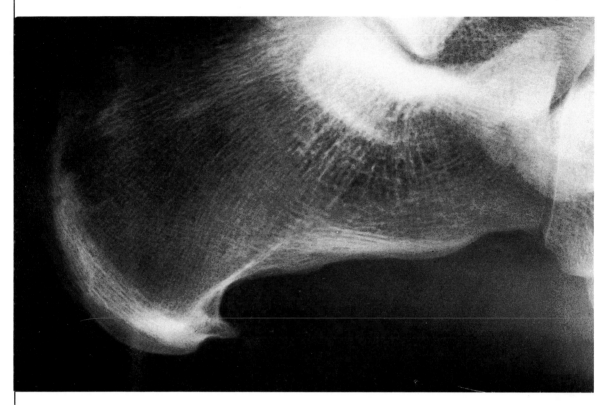

Figure 12.16. (Above). Lateral view of the heel of an athlete with a history suggestive of plantar fascitis.

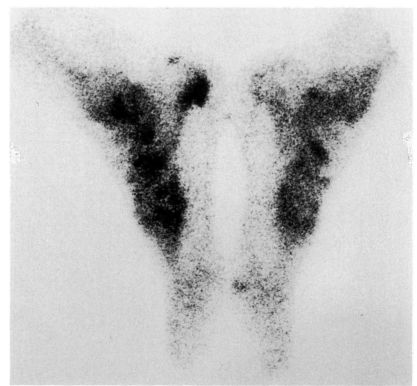

Figure 12.17. (Right). Bone scan of the same patient as illustrated in Figure 12.16 showing an area of increased activity in the left foot related to the calcaneal spur.

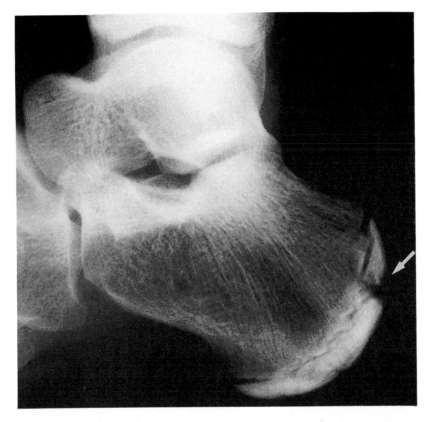

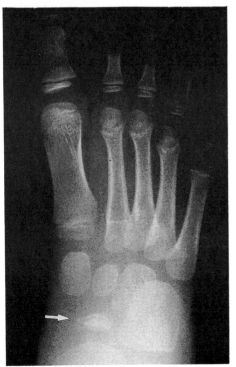

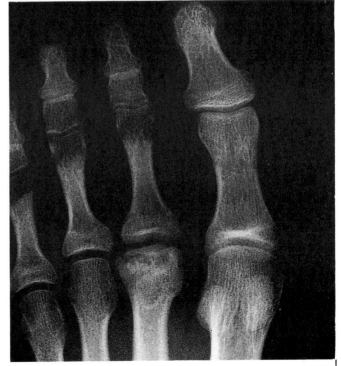

Figure 12.18. (Left). Lateral view of the heel of a 12-year-old girl showing a sclerotic and fragmented calcaneal apophysis (Sever's disease). These appearances would be regarded as unremarkable in the absence of symptoms.

Figure 12.19. (Below left). Plain X-ray of the right foot of a six-year-old dancer demonstrating the classical appearances of osteochondritis of the navicular (Kohler's disease) which is sclerotic and compressed.

Figure 12.20. (Below right). X-ray of the foot of an 18-year-old dancer demonstrating osteochondritis of the head of the second metatarsal (Freiberg's infraction).

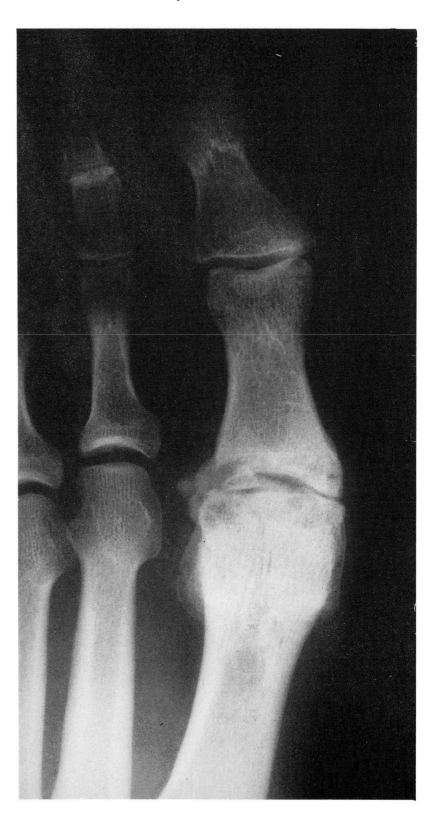

Figure 12.21. X-ray of the left first metatarsophalangeal joint in a 30-year-old ballet dancer showing gross osteoarthritis secondary to repeated 'trauma'.

● BIBLIOGRAPHY ●

Bernstein, A. and Stone, J. R. (1944) March fracture. A report of three hundred and seven cases and a new method of treatment. *J. Bone Joint Surg.* **26**, 743.

Bertram, D. R. (1944) 'Stress' fracture of bone. *Br. J. Radiol.* **17**, 257.

Cailliet, R. (1968) *Foot and Ankle Pain.* Philadelphia: Davis Company.

Childress, H. M. (1943) March fractures of the lower extremity. Report of a case of march fracture of a cuneiform bone. *War Med.* **4**, 152.

Darby, R. E. (1967) Stress fractures of the os calcis. *J. Am. Med. Ass.* **200**, 1183.

Delee, J. C., Evans, J. P. and Julian, J. (1983) Stress fracture of the fifth metatarsal. *Am. J. Sports Med.* **5**, 349.

Devas, M. B. (1963) Stress fractures in children. *J. Bone Joint Surg.* **45(B)**, 528.

Devas, M. B. (1975) *Stress Fractures:* New York: Churchill Livingstone.

Eichenboltz, S. N. and Levine, D. B. (1964) Fractures of the tarsal navicular bone. *Clin. Orthop.* **34**, 142.

Ferguson, A. B. and Gingrich, R. M. (1957) The normal and abnormal calcaneal apophysis and tarsal navicular. *Clin. Orthop.* **10**, 87.

Fowler, A. and Phillip, J. F. (1945) Abnormality of calcaneus as a cause of painful heel: its diagnosis and operative treatment. *Br. J. Surg.* **32**, 494.

Freiberg, A. H. (1914) Infraction of the second metatarsal bone: a typical injury. *Surg. Gynecol. Obstet.* **19**, 191.

Galasko, C. S. B. and Weber, D. A. (eds) (1984) *Radionuclide Scintigraphy in Orthopaedics. Current Problems in Orthopaedics.* Edinburgh: Churchill Livingstone.

Gilbert, R. S. and Johnson, H. A. (1966) Stress fractures in military recruits—a review of twelve years' experience. *Milit. Med.* **131**, 716.

Goergen, T. G., Venn-Watson, E. A., Rossman, D. J., Resnick, D. and Gerber, K. H. (1981) Tarsal navicular fractures in runners. *Am. J. Roentgenol.* **136**, 201.

Graham, C. E. (1970) Stress fractures in joggers. *Texas Med. J.* **66**, 68.

Hartley, J. B. (1943) 'Stress' or 'fatigue' fractures in bone. *Br. J. Radiol.* **16**, 255.

Hullinger, C. W. (1944) Insufficiency fracture of the calcaneus similar to march fracture of metatarsal. *J. Bone Joint Surg.* **26**, 751.

Hunter, L. Y. (1981) Stress fracture of the tarsal navicular. *Am. J. Sports Med.* **9**, 217.

Jones, R. (1901) Fracture of the base of the fifth metatarsal bone by indirect violence. *Ann. Surg.* **35**, 697.

Kohler, A. (1908) Über eine haufige bisher anscheinend unbekannte Erkrankung einszelner kindlicher Knochen. *Munchener Medizinische Wochenschrift* **55**, 923.

LeVeau, B. (1977) *Williams and Lissner. Biomechanics of Human Motion*, 2nd edn. Philadelphia: W. B. Saunders.

McBryde, A. M. (1975) Stress fractures in athletes. *J. Sports Med.* **3(5)**, 212.

McBryde, A. M. (1985) Stress fractures in runners. *Clin. Sports Med.* **4**, 737.

McKenzie, D. C., Taunton, J. E., Clement, D. B., *et al.* (1981) Calcaneal epiphysitis in young athletes. *Can. J. Appl. Sport Sci.* **6**, 123.

Maurice, H. D., Newman, J. H. and Watt, I. (1987) Bone scanning of the foot for unexplained pain. *J. Bone Joint Surg.* **69(B)**, 448.

Nordentoft, J. M. (1940) Some cases of soldier's fracture. *Acta Radiol.* **21**, 615.

Orava, S., Puranen, J. and Ala-Kwetola, L. (1978) Stress fractures caused by physical exercise. *Acta Orth. Scand.* **49**, 19.

Pappas, A. M. (1967) The osteochondroses. *Pediatr. Clin. N. Am.* **14**, 549.

Pavlov, H., Torg, J. S. and Freiberger, R. H. (1983) Tarsal navicular stress fractures: radiographic evaluation. *Radiology* **148**, 641.

Prather, J. L., Nusynowitz, M. L., Snowdy, H. A., *et al.* (1977) Scintigraphic findings in stress fractures. *J. Bone Joint Surg.* **59(A)**, 869.

Renstrom, P. and Johnson, R. J. (1985) Over-use injuries in sports: a review. *Sports Med.* **2**, 316.

Santopietro, F. J. (1988) Foot and foot related injuries in the young athlete. *Clin. Sports Med.* **7(3)**, 563.

Sever, J. W. (1912) Apophysitis of the os calcis. *N.Y. Med. J.* **95**, 1025.

Sewell, J. R., Black, C. M., Chapman, A. H., *et al.* (1980) Quantitative scintigraphy in diagnosis and management of plantar fascitis (calcaneal periostitis): concise communications. *J. Nucl. Med.* **21**, 633.

Smillie, I. S. (1957) Freiberg's infraction. *J. Bone Joint Surg.* **39(B)**, 580.

13 Soft Tissue Injuries

Soft tissue injuries occur frequently in sports of all kinds and the vast majority are quickly self-resolving, although some can become chronic problems. Conventional radiology and bone scanning have been of little value in these conditions, and CT scanning has not helped in the majority of cases. However, the advent of high quality ultrasound scans has made a major contribution by demonstrating fluid collections and muscle tears. Ultrasound has the advantage of being relatively readily available and, because there is no problem with ionizing radiation, the resolution of the lesion can be followed and the examination can be repeated as often as necessary. More recently the appearance of MRI scanning, which appears to be even more sensitive, has aided diagnosis in difficult cases where it now appears to be the investigation of choice.

Haematomas and muscle ruptures in the thigh can be readily delineated using ultrasound, and the quadriceps femoris is particularly easy to scan, as is shown in Figure 13.1. The normal anatomy can be well demonstrated, as can large fluid collections due to bleeding; with experience, complete muscle tears can be shown. The injury illustrated here was sustained by a 24-year-old soccer player who kicked the ground instead of the ball.

Occasionally such muscle damage progresses into myositis ossificans, the patient presenting with recurrent muscle tears. Fortunately this is an uncommon complication as it is often difficult to treat. The soft tissue ossification is readily seen on ultrasound as an echodense lesion casting an acoustic shadow as shown in Figure 13.2, where there is a long linear area of myositis ossificans lying in the quadriceps of a 20-year-old rugby player. This area can be examined with conventional radiology, and the abnormality confirmed as shown in Figure 13.3. In this condition there is active calcium deposition which results in abnormal activity on isotope bone scanning. The abnormal area is often much larger than suspected, with increased pick-up extending over a wide area as shown in Figure 13.4. The demonstration of continuing activity may be helpful in the assessment and subsequent management of the clinical problem.

MRI scanning is also extremely sensitive in demonstrating muscle

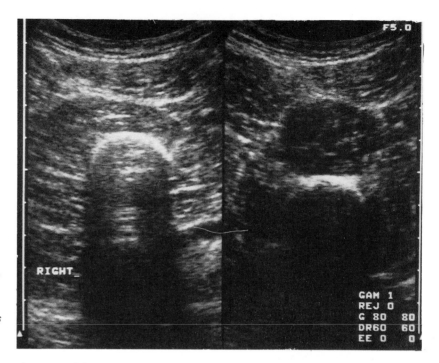

Figure 13.1. Transverse ultrasound scan of the quadriceps femoris region. The right side is normal. On the left side there is discontinuity of the muscle with a large, less sonorich area representing a haematoma.

damage with its associated bleeding, and it can also distinguish between old and new problems. Figure 13.5 is an MRI scan of the thighs demonstrating both a recent and an older haematoma on the left.

Injuries to the calf are common, and athletes are not always sure whether they have received a direct blow to the area or whether the pain is the result of a tear occurring when a sudden severe strain was placed on the muscle. Ultrasound can again prove useful in this region but, where available, MRI scanning gives more information. Figure 13.6 is a typical case where transverse scans of the calves have been performed. The left side is quite normal and there is clearly a collection of fluid due to a resolving haematoma lying between the muscle planes of the right calf in this 34-year-old cricketer. The muscles themselves appear intact.

When dealing with acute problems in the region of the tendo-Achilles it can sometimes be difficult to decide whether there has been a complete tear of the tendon, a partial tear with a haematoma or, in chronic cases, whether this is just a stress phenomenon at the insertion of the tendon into the calcaneus. Localized X-rays of the heel occasionally help although usually, as in Figure 13.7, the changes are minimal. Where the plain films are thought to be equivocal an isotope bone scan will confirm the presence of abnormal activity (Figure 13.8), due to an apophysitis in this young athlete.

Demonstration of the tendo-Achilles itself can be readily performed using suitable ultrasound scanning techniques. A normal tendon is clearly shown as a sonolucent linear shadow, on the left in Figure 13.9. The presence of haematomas and incomplete tears show as areas of increased shadowing within the tendon sheath, as seen on the right in this examination of a 19-year-old soccer player. By asking the athlete to contract the relevant muscles during the examination the presence of complete tears can be confirmed, although the total disruption may often be readily seen without active movements, as in this young sprinter (Figure 13.10).

Similarly MRI scanning also demonstrates ruptures and haematomas in the tendo-Achilles very readily (Figure 13.11), as we see in this illustration of a late presenting tear on the left.

We feel that, where it is thought that imaging will help confirm a diagnosis, the investigation of first choice is an ultrasound scan of the area performed by an experienced ultrasonographer. Only if this fails to demonstrate the problem do we consider referring the patient for MRI scans—mainly for reasons of availability and cost. We occasionally use isotope bone scanning techniques and conventional films, although generally we do not find these particularly helpful.

Figure 13.2. (Below left). Longitudinal ultrasound scan of the thigh. There is an echodense lesion in the muscle casting a shadow, this is an area of myositis ossificans.

Figure 13.3. (Below right). Localized magnified X-ray of the thigh of the case shown in Figure 13.2. The area of myositis ossificans is shown (arrow).

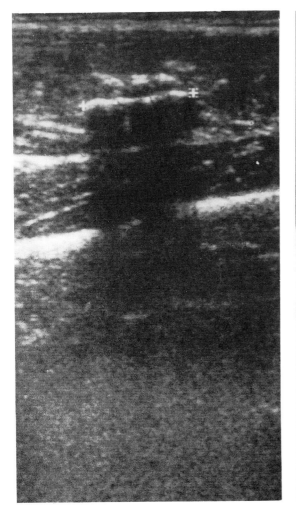

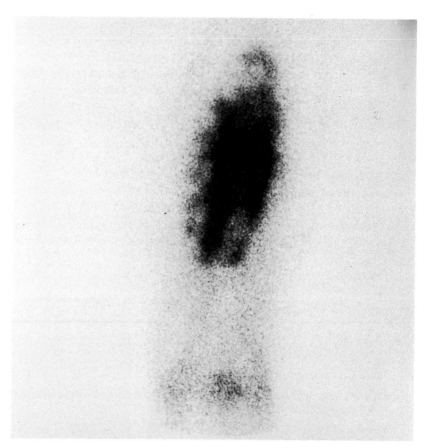

Figure 13.4. Isotope bone scan of the thigh (of the case shown in Figures 13.2 and 13.3), indicating that the abnormal area is very extensive and that the myositis ossificans is 'active'.

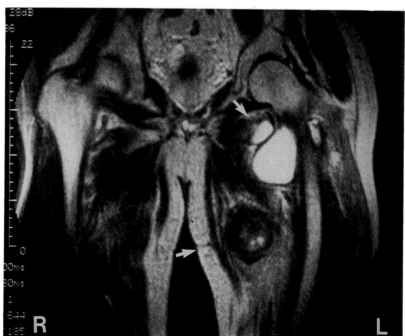

Figure 13.5. Longitudinal coronal MRI scan of the thighs. The right side is normal. There are old and new haematomas demonstrated on the left side, lying medial to the femur (arrows).

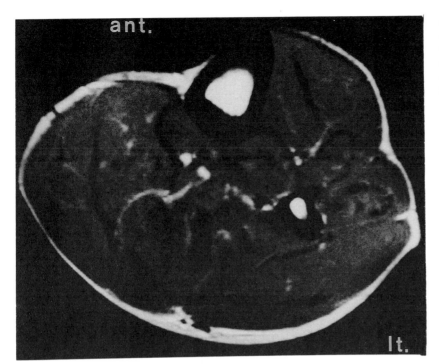

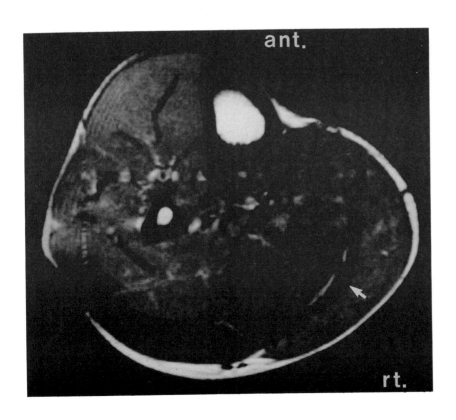

Figure 13.6. Transverse MRI scan of the legs. The left side is normal. There is a resolving haematoma on the right side lying posteriorly between the muscle planes of the calf.

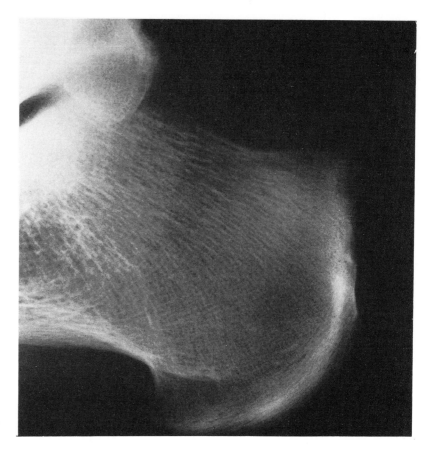

Figure 13.7. Lateral X-ray of the heel. There is some irregularity and sclerosis posteriorly.

Figure 13.8. Isotope bone scan of the case shown in Figure 13.7 confirming that the irregular area is abnormal with marked activity at the site of the tendo-Achilles insertion.

Figure 13.9. (Facing top). Longitudinal ultrasound of the tendo-Achilles. The left side is normal; there is a haematoma and partial tear of the right tendon.

Figure 13.10. (Facing bottom). Longitudinal ultrasound scan of the tendo-Achilles. There is a discontinuity indicating a complete tear, and an associated haematoma lying proximal to the tear in the tendon sheath.

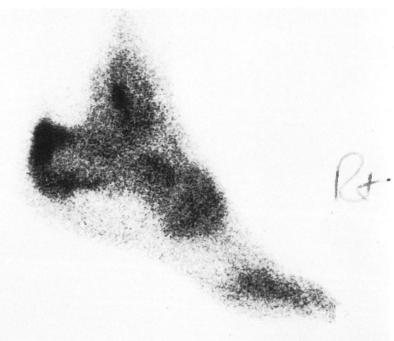

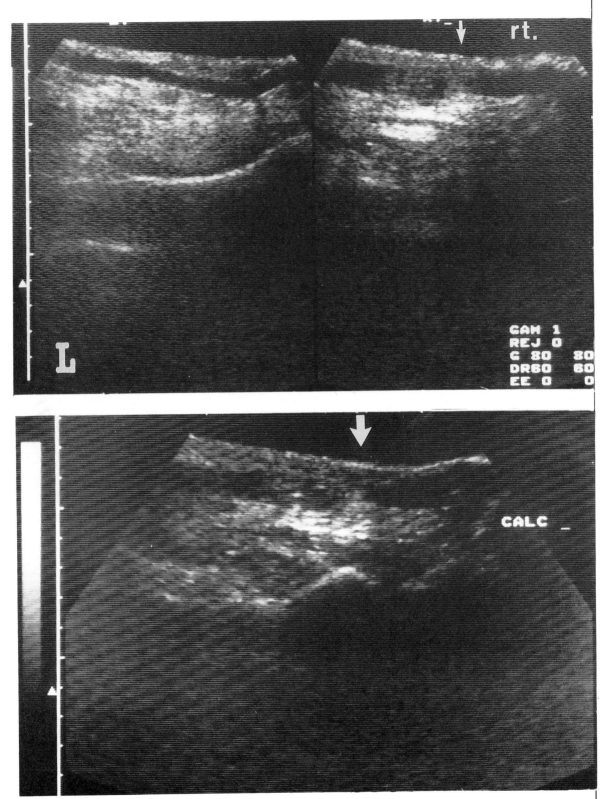

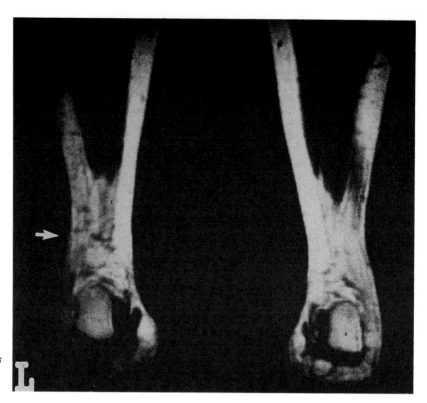

Figure 13.11. Longitudinal coronal MRI scans of the tendo-Achilles. The right side is normal; there is a tear on the left side.

● BIBLIOGRAPHY ●

Ackerman, L. V. (1958) Extra-osseous localized non-neoplastic bone and cartilage formation (so-called myositis ossificans). *J. Bone Joint Surg.* **40(A)**, 279.

Blei, C. L., Nirschl, R. P. and Grant, E. G. (1986) Achilles tendon: U.S. diagnosis of pathologic conditions. *Radiology* **159**, 765.

Cady, E. B., Gardener, J. E. and Edwards, R. H. T. (1983) Ultrasonic tissue characterization of skeletal muscle. *Eur. J. Clin. Invest.* **13**, 469.

Dillehay, G. L., Deschler, T., Rogers, L. F., Neiman, H. L. and Hendrix, R. W. (1984) The ultrasonographic characterization of tendons. *Invest. Radiol.* **19**, 338.

Ehman, R. L., Berquist, T. H. and McLoed, R. A. (1988) M.R. Imaging of the musculo-skeletal system: A five year appraisal. *Radiology* **166**, 313.

Ellis, M. and Frank, H. G. (1966) Myositis ossificans traumatica: with special reference to the quadriceps femoris muscle. *J. Trauma* **6**, 724.

Grindrod, S., Tofts, P. and Edwards, R. (1983) Investigation of human skeletal muscle structure and composition by X-ray computerized tomography. *Eur. J. Clin. Invest.* **13**, 465.

Jackson, D. W. and Feagin, J. A. (1973) Quadriceps contusions in young athletes. *J. Bone Joint Surg.* **55(A)**, 95.

Kleinmann, M. and Gross, A. E. (1983) Achilles tendon rupture following steroid injection. *J. Bone Joint Surg.* **65(A)**, 1345.

Kramer, F. L., Kurtz, A. B., Rubin, C. and Goldberg, B. B. (1979) Ultrasound appearance of myositis ossificans. *Skeletal Radiol.* **4**, 19.

Kuwada, G. T. and Schuberth, J. (1984) Evaluation of Achilles tendon rerupture. *J. Foot Surg.* **23**, 340.

Laine, H. R., Harjula, A. L. J. and Peltokallio, P. (1987) Ultrasonography as a differential diagnostic aid in achillodynia. *J. Ultrasound Med.* **6**, 351.

Leach, R. E., James, S. and Wasilewski, S. (1982) Achilles tendinitis. *Am. J. Sports Med.* **9**, 93.

Leonardi, M., Ulivi, M. and Balconi, M. (1983) Echotomography in sports traumatology. *Sports Traum.* **4**, 49.

Maffulli, N., *et al.* (1987) Ultrasound diagnosis of Achilles tendon pathology in runners. *Brit. J. Sports Med.* **21**, 158.

Mathieson, J. R., *et al.* (1988) Sonography of the Achilles tendon and adjacent bursae. *Am. J. Roentgenol.* **151**, 127.

Mayer, R. and Wilhelm, K. J. (1984) Sonography of Achilles tendon rupture. *Digitale Bild-diagn.* **4**, 185.

Milgram, J. E. (1953) Muscle ruptures and avulsions with particular reference to the lower extremities. *AAOS Instructional Course Lectures* **10**, 233.

Moon, K. L., *et al.* (1983) Musculoskeletal applications of nuclear magnetic resonance. *Radiology* **147**, 161.

Puddu, G., Ippolito, E. and Postacchini, F. (1976) A classification of Achilles tendon disease. *Am. J. Sports Med.* **4**, 145.

Quinn, S. F., Murray, W. T., Clark, R. A. and Cochran, C. F. (1987) Achilles tendon: M.R. Imaging at 1.5T. *Radiology* **164**, 767.

Scheller, A. D., Kasser, J. R. and Quigley, T. B. (1980) Tendon injuries about the ankle. *Symp. Sports Inj.* **2**, 801.

Smart, G. W., Taunton, J. E. and Clement, D. B. (1980) Achilles tendon disorders in runners. A review. *Med. Sci. Sports Exercise* **12**, 231.

Vazelle, F., Roland, J. J., Rochcongen, P. and Ramee, A. (1982) Contribution à l'analyse de l'image radiologique du tendon d'Achille. Étude radio-echoanatomique. Localization du plantaire grele. *J. Radiol.* (France) **65**, 351.

Zeanah, W. R. and Hudson, T. M. (1982) Myositis ossificans. Radiologic evaluation of two cases with diagnostic computed tomograms. *Clin. Orthop.* **168**, 187.

Index

Figures in *italic* type